D0855967

METABOLICS

METABOLICS

Putting Your Food Energy to Work

LAWRENCE E. LAMB, M.D.

HARPER & ROW, PUBLISHERS

New York, Evanston, San Francisco, London

Designed by Janice Stern

Library of Congress Cataloging in Publication Data

Lamb, Lawrence E
    Metabolics: putting your food energy to work.
    1. Nutrition. 2. Metabolism. I. Title. [DNLM: 1. Food—Popular works.
2. Metabolism—Popular works. 3. Nutrition—Popular works. QU120 L218m]
QP141.L16   612'.39   74-1829
ISBN 0-06-012484-9

ACKNOWLEDGMENTS

It's not easy to present complex material on what human cells do with the food we eat simply enough for the general public to grasp the main principles involved. By using simplified block arrangements I have attempted to present this material so that anyone who can stack blocks together can follow what happens.

The biochemist will just have to live with these simplifications for the lay reader. I have rearranged the structure of water for example, to HHO as opposed to HOH. This will help the reader without a chemistry background. Those knowledgeable enough to know that I have made these rearrangements should also be able to adapt to the presentation.

All of the basic factual material in the book on how the body processes food is based on a wide variety of standard and well-accepted physiology, biochemistry, and pharmacology texts. The food values are based on data from the U.S. Department of Agriculture.

I want to take this opportunity to express my appreciation to Joyce Boston and Vivian Lindsey of the San Antonio, Texas, Manpower, Inc. office for typing the manuscript, and their patience with my many alterations. Their capable efforts made the job much easier.

L.E.L.

CONTENTS

1 It's About Energy   1

2 What's Really in Your Food   7

3 Getting It to Your Energy Cells   13

4 Your Energy Shuttle   20

5 What Are Carbohydrates?   28

6 Getting Energy from Carbohydrates   39

7 What Are Fats?   47

8 Fat to Energy, Energy to Fat   58

9 What Are Proteins?   67

10 Proteins: How Much? What Kind? Where to Get Them?   77

11 How You Use Proteins   86

12 Getting Energy from Alcohol   97

13 Putting Your Energy System Together   104

14 Do You Need Choline and Lecithin?   111

15 Controlling Your Blood Sugar   114

16 Why Diabetics Are Tired   123

17 Low Blood Sugar and Your Energy   131

18 Your Energy System Needs Vitamins   140

19 Vitamin B_1, Thiamine   145

20 Vitamin B_2, Riboflavin   150

21 Niacin   153

22   Pantothenic Acid   158

23   Vitamin B_6, Pyridoxine   161

24   Vitamin B_{12}, Cyanocobalamin   163

25   Folic Acid and PABA   166

26   Biotin and Inositol   168

27   Vitamin C, Ascorbic Acid   170

28   Vitamin A   176

29   Vitamin E   182

30   Vitamin K   187

31   Vitamin D   188

32   It Takes Calcium and Phosphorus Too   191

33   The Truth About Magnesium   197

34   Why You Need Iron, Manganese, Cobalt, and Copper   200

35   Iodine and Your Thyroid   205

36   You Need Salt and Water   210

37   How to Plan a Healthy Diet   216

38   Undernutrition Robs Your Energy   230

39   Those Fad Weight-Reducing Methods Can Be a Drag   237

40   Sensible Weight Control to Protect Your Health and
     Energy Level   245

     Index   259

1

IT'S ABOUT ENERGY

Do you have enough energy? Or does that old tired feeling keep you from really enjoying life because you lack energy? Many people have this problem because they don't understand metabolics, the basis for healthy eating and living patterns.

Everyone talks about diets. Book after book is written on what you should eat. There are innumerable diets to lose weight—most of them unsound—and diets for "low blood sugar," diabetes, gout, and other problems. You can read that sugar is bad for you, almost a terrible poison, or that fats should be avoided. You can read any number of accounts extolling the virtues of a variety of vitamins and minerals. What is missing is factual information about what the body does with food after you eat it. This, of course, is the basis for deciding what you should eat, which foods are good for you, and which are bad.

Doctors call the study of what the body does with foods metabolism. This is why I have called this book *Metabolics*. The word comes from the Greek *metabolos*, which means changeable. That is what metabolics is all about: how the body changes, literally by using energy and chemicals from food to build body structures.

Metabolics involves one of the most fascinating processes of nature— the process in which the steak you eat, or the piece of pie, is converted into simple chemicals within the cells. Part of the food can be used to release energy for body functions. Most of this energy is not used for physical work. That may surprise you since in weight control there is so much emphasis on the relationship of physical activity to calories eaten. A lot of the energy in your food will be used to build new compounds and, more important, to move uncountable numbers of chemicals into and out of your active cells.

The most active cells are not fat cells, incidentally. Every cell in your body is a chemical processing plant. There is a processing unit to tear down chemicals and another unit to assemble new compounds, such as proteins, for enzymes and hormones. Chemicals must be carried into the cell and the end products transported out of the cell. This constant massive migration requires energy. It does not occur by simple diffusion, like salt dissolving in water. Every cell that forms an enzyme or hormone to be used elsewhere in the body must provide the energy to move its newly formed chemical out of the cell. Even moving food particles across the cell membrane in the intestine requires energy. This has a lot to do with why you need energy, even if you are just resting. Your vital cell processing plant simply can't work without energy.

Energy is also needed to build new body structures, the process that keeps you young. The steak you eat contains proteins. These are made up of those important amino acids. The amino acids are the building blocks used by the body to manufacture new proteins. It takes energy to hook one amino-acid unit to another, much as heat energy is used to weld two pieces of metal together. You need energy to grow a new hair, replace those skin cells that are constantly flaking off, or grow those astonishing 200 million new red blood cells each minute. Not only do you lose cells from the outer surface of your body, but the cells lining your digestive tract are also constantly shedding. The small intestine alone is claimed to shed over a half pound of cells a day. It completely renews itself every three days. This is quite a replacement act. True, you can reuse the energy that evolves from the breakdown of the old red cells and internal structures (but not from those outer surface structures such as hair, nails, and skin), but with each transformation there is a loss of some energy. The process isn't perfect, but then few things are.

Food, then, must provide the building blocks for new body structures, as well as the energy to do the building. You can see there is a lot of truth to that old saying, "You are what you eat." When food is not used for energy or as building blocks it is converted to a storage form for future use. A small amount is stored as animal starch, called "glycogen," and the rest as fat. The body makes no distinction as to whether the food is fat, carbohydrate, protein, or even alcohol. If there are excess food products available after the small amount of glycogen is formed, they will all be converted to fat. That's right, protein you don't need for building or energy is just another way of increasing your fat deposits.

The body has a remarkable processing plant. It can take the wide variety of foods we eat and convert them to a few simple compounds that eventually are processed in the same way. It is this remarkable ability of the body to simplify the process that makes metabolics a fairly simple concept. If you can count, you can follow what happens to the food you eat. Just as you can use wood, coal, gas, or electricity to produce heat, the body can use fats, carbohydrates, or proteins to produce energy. When you see how the body does this you can begin to understand—and make some value judgments about—some diet fads. You can see for yourself the truth about the constantly recycled low-carbohydrate diet fads and other so-called "health miracles."

If you are overweight you need to know just what your body does with the food you eat. This is the only way you can understand what you need to do about your eating habits. It seems like almost everyone is on a diet for something, usually to lose weight. If you are one of those people, you may be sapping your energy. What's worse, the diet, if successful, may make it more difficult for you to avoid getting fat in the future. Does that sound like a startling statement to you? It should. The public has been brainwashed for years to diet to lose weight, or to "burn off those calories" with exercise. If you are like many thousands of moderately overweight people, you may not need to do either. And doing it may actually be dangerous.

I want to introduce you to an exciting new way to do something constructive about your weight. Rather than talk about treating the symptoms of being "overweight," I would like to explain the most common cause of obesity in our society and what to do about it. The result will give you a lot more energy, and you will feel better without going on a highly restricted diet that may harm you. You should know from the beginning that there is an alternative to starving yourself or spending hours and hours sweating off calories. The facts are all there. I am not proposing anything that has not already been established by medical science, if you take the time to look at the facts. The facts have been largely ignored because of the overemphasis on semistarvation diets and on the number of calories used in specific physical activities. That is only part of the story. The rest of the story is what happens while you are resting. That's right, the calories your body uses when you are not doing anything. Let me tell you at once I am not proposing that calories don't count, or any other weirdo concept. I'm talking about a sound, scientific approach to the cause of obesity and what to do about it. In some instances a diet plan is necessary. Physical activity is important because it uses calories, but there is much more to the metabolic scheme of things than only this.

The calories you use at rest are the overhead expense of running your body. The calories you eat are your total income of energy. The calories you use in physical activity are taken from those left after the overhead-calorie expense. Any calories that are left over after both overhead and spending are stored as fat. The problem in a nutshell is that scientists have too long looked only at the calories-in and the calories-spent. Almost no attention has been given to the overhead-calories, or how many calories you use at rest. And they are quite important, as you will see as you study the information about what your body does with food. Can you imagine any company's budget working by considering the money in (gross income) and the profit to spend (net) with no consideration of the overhead cost? That is about what most people are told in regard to obesity. The treatment is usually the same, "eat less," by whatever means or gimmick, or "exercise more" to spend those calories. Have you ever heard anyone tell you to do something about your body so that you use more calories at rest? I suspect not.

If you are underweight—or think you are—you also need to understand the role food plays in gaining weight, particularly if you want to grow bone and muscle instead of fat.

A host of mistaken ideas are accepted by the public daily because they do not understand what the body does with food. Many swallow various food preparations and supplements in the hopes that these will impart a greater level of health or energy. One of the most common mistaken ideas is that if you eat something it will increase the amount of this substance in the body. It is not true that eating lots of meat will put more meat on your bones. It may put some fat around them, but don't expect to grow any new muscles just by eating. Many people waste their money on protein supplements because they do not understand what determines how much protein they need. The never-ending prescription of pills, powders, natural foods, quick energy compounds, natural vitamins, and combinations of miracle minerals is not far removed from the odious practices of medical charlatans who peddled "snake oil" cures to their true believers. We still think that eating certain substances imparts high levels of health and vigor—just as some primitive peoples ate parts of their relatives or even enemies to gain strength or desired traits.

Some of the health substances are helpful to some people with health problems. It is true that if you are on a protein-deficient diet and fail to get your needed protein from common food, protein supplements will be helpful. It is equally true that if you have a vitamin deficiency, regardless of the cause, taking vitamins will work miraculous results.

Energy can be improved by improving your diet, if it needs improving. Our sense of energy and well-being is dependent on the release of energy within the cells. This requires not only the right food elements, but also adequate delivery of oxygen to the cells to accomplish the important metabolic changes. Individuals with poor circulation, lung disease, or anemia severe enough to limit the oxygen delivery, all experience fatigue. All these conditions can hinder the cells from getting the vital chemicals from the food and the oxygen needed to release food energy.

Symptomatic of the general lack of understanding about food and what the body does with it is the habit of saying that a substance is bad because "it's chemical." No foods, additives, minerals, or other substances are good or bad simply because they are chemicals. All foods are chemicals. Our entire body is chemical. All the things we know are either chemical or related to chemicals. The entire earth and its environment is made of little more than a hundred chemical elements. To stop eating because something is chemical is to stop eating entirely.

Not far behind the fads to lose weight are many prevalent ideas about low blood sugar. This has become a popular diagnosis for all those ill-defined feelings many people have—with or without any laboratory measurements to confirm it. Diets for this problem, real or fancied, run the gamut of the imaginations of physicians and nonphysicians alike. Some eat a diet almost devoid of carbohydrates, and the miraculous body simply maintains the blood sugar (glucose) by converting proteins to glucose. The cells still need energy, and they will simply use proteins and fat for this purpose. Some of the cells of our nervous system and some other cells require glucose for energy and cannot survive without it.

Those who do have medical problems related to diet can profit from understanding what the body does about food. This includes the diabetic, the overweight, the underweight, those with thyroid disorders, and all those who have, or think they have, low blood sugar. In addition, all people who are smart enough to realize that to stay healthy they must eat right need to understand the concept of metabolics.

Growth can be affected by what you eat, and the reason for this is explained by metabolics. It is no accident that Japanese children are much larger since they have changed former diet practices. The children of postwar Japan outgrew their parents so fast that they were unable to use the same school furniture that had been used for generations.

There is a difference in the kind of proteins you eat. You can stunt a child's growth or impair an adult's health if there are not sufficient amounts of the right proteins in the food he eats. And it matters whether your calories are liquid or solid, fat or carbohydrates, and even hot or cold.

Those new food labels will mean a lot more to you when you understand how the body processes the food. Anyone who has shopped in a grocery store and read the labels has been confronted with such terms as "monoglycerides," "diglycerides," "triglycerides," "hardened," and "partially hydrogenated." What difference does it make? Your key to understanding and using the information available to you about food is understanding your body. That means understanding metabolics. How well you succeed in this may determine how much energy you have and how healthy you really are.

2

WHAT'S REALLY IN YOUR FOOD

We need to look at just what food and drink contain. All those innumerable dishes are composed of a limited number of basic parts. Of course, the beverages contain water, but did you know that meat, fish, vegetables, and fruit also contain large amounts of water? A pound of raw lean round steak with the fat removed contains about three-fourths of a pint of water. Over 70 per cent of its weight is water. About 5 per cent of its weight is fat, and that represents over 30 per cent of its calories. The nutrients in most of our common foods in their natural state are diluted with water. Beefsteak, then, is actually a small amount of protein and fat diluted with a large amount of water. Don't be too surprised, for more than half of your own body is water.

You should learn to think of the water in the food you eat. This has a lot to do with how many calories there are in a given food. Lean round steak is a good item on a reducing diet, not because protein is so much better for you than carbohydrates for this purpose, but because lean steak has a low calorie value for its weight and bulk. A whole pound of lean round steak contains only 600 calories. Fish and poultry are also low-calorie foods because of their water content.

Many foods are high in calories because they contain little or no water. Butter and margarine are good examples. Only 20 per cent of the weight of these products is water, and that is about the same percentage of water you find in the fat around the meat you eat. The low percentage of water is the main reason why fat foods contain so many calories. Besides, a gram of fat contains over twice as many calories as a gram of either carbohydrates or proteins. Table sugar contains less than 0.5 per cent water. That's pretty dry, and, of course, it gets that way by processing it from its natural source in the beet or cane. A small amount of sugar contains a lot of calories primarily because it is undiluted by water. This is also true of flour. Lard is one of the highest calorie foods since it contains no water and is all fat. A pound of lard (4,091 calories) contains almost seven times as many calories as a pound of the separable lean of round steak.

The food value in many items, particularly vegetables, fruit, and cereals, is diluted by the indigestible fibrous material they contain. This is cellulose, and in our digestive system it is treated as an inert object, just as plain cotton would be. Some animals can process cellulose because of special features in their digestive system (for example, the cow, with her four stomachs). The cellulose and the water content of many vegetables make them relatively low-calorie foods.

The fibrous material serves an important purpose: it provides the bulk in the diet necessary for the normal movement of the food and waste through the digestive system. Some authorities believe that cereal fiber, in particular, is important to normal bowel function. They believe the high incidence of cancer of the bowel seen in the United States, England, Canada, and other industrialized nations (the highest rate in the world is in New England) is a direct consequence of not eating sufficient amounts of whole-cereal fibers. This happens because people tend to eat foods made with refined flour from which the cereal fiber has been removed. To counteract this problem experts advise eating at least a cup of bran a day and making an effort to eat foods made with whole cereals.

Cellulose is really a carbohydrate, and I'll say more about that when we discuss carbohydrates. It is a plant product, not found in animal foods. You can think of it as the skeleton of the plants, since it supplies the tough fibrous material that gives a plant its shape.

Carbohydrates are a main source of food energy. Primitive man may have existed entirely on carbohydrates, at least for long periods of time. As historian H. G. Wells has pointed out, primitive man was a small creature, unable to cope with the wild beasts of his time, such as the giant mammoth and bear. He was more likely to be "the hunted rather than the hunter." This limited rather sharply his opportunities to be a carnivore. Like other primates, primitive man had the grinding teeth of vegetarians, rather than the overriding teeth of the carnivore. Many naturalists believe that early man was essentially a vegetarian, particularly in the jungle and rain-forest environments. A casual perusal of history reveals that even northern European man had abundant sources of carbohydrates. The earliest primitive drawings show men taking wild honey from the bees, and they had a kind of mead they made from a mixture of honey and berry juice.

Some of the popular low-carbohydrate books, notably *Dr. Atkins' Diet Revolution* and *Calories Don't Count*, have claimed that man originally did not eat carbohydrates, and, hence, his body is really not suited to processing any large amounts of carbohydrates. Nothing could be further from the truth. Quite the contrary, primitive man was not accustomed to eating meat. As soon as man began to develop civilizations he began to cultivate cereals, vegetables, and fruits. As long ago as 4000 B.C. the natives of Mohenjo Daro, an area now known as Pakistan, were irrigating their crops, and carbohydrates were a mainstay of their diet.

It should be emphasized that carbohydrates are a natural food for man. In many societies where they account for over 80 per cent of the calories eaten, the people are healthy, robust, and free of many of our medical problems, such as heart disease, diabetes, "low blood sugar," obesity, and bowel problems. So don't be fooled by misinformation. Man naturally eats carbohydrates.

The foods that contain the greatest proportion of carbohydrates are vegetables, fruits, legumes or mature bean seeds, cereals, nuts, melons, and berries. Obviously, these are also the foods that provide many of our needed vitamins and the bulk for our diet. You will also find carbohydrates in milk and milk products. Then there are the refined carbohydrates, which include sugar, honey, syrups, and molasses. Some would include white flour in this category, too. It makes a difference whether the carbohydrate comes from one of the sweets or from a natural product like vegetables. Your body may respond differently to them, and you will learn why when you read how the body processes carbohydrates.

There is a surprising amount of fat in your food. You can see the fat around the muscle fibers of the meat, but did you know that there is a lot more invisible fat within the muscle fibers? Of course, the most tender steaks are the ones that contain the most hidden fat. There is also a lot of fat in homemade or bakery cakes, with a few exceptions like angel-food cakes. There is as much fat in many rich devil's-food cakes as there is in a fairly fat steak. Sweet rolls, pie crust, and many other baked products are loaded with fat. There is also some fat in raw fruit. A lot of the so-called low-fat foods are really low-calorie foods with a reasonable percentage of their total calories as fat.

You will want to understand a lot about fat, because so much is said about fats and health. It's important to understand the difference between the saturated fats and the two types of unsaturated fats, monounsaturated and polyunsaturated. There is a lot of evidence that too much fat of any kind in the diet, and particularly too much saturated fat (mostly from animal sources and coconut oil), will increase the likelihood of heart and vascular disease. These lead to heart attacks, strokes, and many other problems. There's no requirement for any major amount of fat in the diet. There is some evidence that you need a very small amount of some of the polyunsaturated fats. And you will need some fat to absorb the fat-soluble vitamins. But that doesn't require very much fat. You won't be able to avoid eating some fat, even if you eat a diet restricted to fruit, vegetables, and cereal. I'm not recommending you do that.

The main purpose of fats in the diet is to provide a concentrated source of calories. If you are a heavy laborer, these might be very useful. If you are an office worker or a housewife, your calorie needs won't be very great.

There is a great deal of confusion about cholesterol. It is not a fat, although eating too much fat induces the body to produce excess amounts of cholesterol. It contains no calories. Technically, it is an alcohol. It is a waxy substance formed chiefly by the liver, and it is relatively insoluble. It is carried by the bile into the intestine. The fatty particles that lodge in the arteries of the body to produce atherosclerosis (which leads to heart attacks, strokes, and other problems) contain lots of cholesterol. Only animal foods contain cholesterol. Plants do not form cholesterol. Saturated fats seem to increase the formation of cholesterol in the body. This is why coconut oil, which is high in saturated fats, should not be used in the diet. It stimulates the body to form too much cholesterol, but it does not contain any cholesterol itself. The main sources of cholesterol are egg yolks and organ meats. There is also some in mammal meat, fish, poultry, milk, and milk products.

Of course, a healthy diet will also include adequate amounts of protein. For most normal adults this will not need to be more than 70 grams a day (400 calories of protein). Protein is found in meat, milk, eggs, cereal, nuts, mature bean seeds, and in small amounts in vegetables.

Many of the foods you have been told are high-protein foods are also high-fat foods. Whole milk is a good example. About half its calories are from fat, some from carbohydrates, and only 23 per cent from protein. The same is true of many meats. If there is much fat on the meat, there will be more calories from fat than from protein. The difficulty here is that you are used to food content being described in terms of percentage by weight and not in terms of calories. The fat in a piece of lean round steak with all the visible fat removed is only 5 per cent of the total weight. That sounds like a low-fat food item. In truth, because over 70 per cent of the steak's weight is water and because fat contains about twice as many calories as protein, that small amount of fat represents nearly a third of the calories in the piece of raw meat. Those meats that contain even more fat will contain more calories from fat than from protein.

The protein in your food is not used directly in the same form as it occurs in the food. It is broken down into its own building blocks, the amino acids. It is really the amino acids that you need. These are used to build new cells, for growth or replacement of worn or damaged cells, and to manufacture vital body substances. Many of the hormones in the body that must be manufactured for life processes are proteins, as are all the enzymes. Amino acids are vital to the life process.

Protein can also be used for energy. If there is not enough protein in your diet, particularly if a state of starvation or semistarvation exists— and this can occur on some diets—the body will use its protein stores, including the protein in the muscles. This is the reason prisoners of war, those in concentration camps, and others under starvation conditions become so emaciated. The muscle protein replaces the protein that should have been available in the food. You can neither grow nor maintain a healthy body without some protein. But taking more protein than your body needs will not grow more muscles or produce more hormones. It will be converted to carbohydrate and used for energy or stored as fat.

For many people, particularly the "executive drinker," a considerable number of calories are consumed each day as alcohol. This is an excellent example of empty calories. Pure alcohol contains no bulk, no vitamins, no minerals—just calories. There are seven calories in each gram of alcohol. It is one of the caloric substances that is also a drug. A standard cocktail made with a jigger of whiskey (1½ ounces) contains about 100 calories, not counting the sugar, fruit juice, and other ingredients that may be added other than water.

If you have a properly balanced diet, your food will contain sufficient amounts of all the necessary vitamins. The only reason people need vitamin pills is because either their diet is inadequate in this respect or they have a medical problem that requires an additional intake of vitamins. Vitamins are essential to the use of the food elements. The important chemical reactions that extract energy from food are dependent on the action of certain vitamins. Even new cell formation depends on some of them.

A group of chemicals in your food are classified as minerals and electrolytes. Common table salt is one of these. The sodium in salt is a necessary chemical in your body fluids. Normally we have about the same amount of sodium in our body fluids as in sea water. If you have too much sodium, you will retain water to dilute the concentration of sodium in the tissues. This will cause swelling from fluid retention. Many women experience this just before their menstrual periods. Patients with disorders of the kidney, heart, and liver will retain fluid, have swollen extremities, and even experience shortness of breath from fluid retained in the lungs.

Potassium is a mineral, similar in many respects to sodium, found in its greatest concentration within the cells. If you lose too much potassium you will feel tired, your heart may not work as well, and you will have other problems which we will discuss later. A good source of potassium is orange juice. In general, the most abundant sources of potassium are fruits and fruit juices.

Often people must make an effort to get enough calcium in their diet. We lose a certain amount every day, and if we don't take in enough, the bones will begin to decalcify. This will lead to a tendency to fractures, deformities of the spine, and other problems. The most common and best source of calcium is milk. You can use either skim milk, nonfat dry-milk powder, low-fat milk, or whole milk to meet your calcium requirements.

Of course, iron is essential in your diet, and some women in the childbearing years don't get nearly enough. A host of trace metals are also important. I'll explain the minerals more fully in a separate section.

There are a number of additives, dyes, and other substances in foods which are not there for their nutritive value. Some of these have come under attack as possible health hazards. And some of them are. It is a mistake, though, to say they are bad because they are chemicals, or because we haven't sufficient proof they are good, or at least not harmful. All of the vital food components I have mentioned to you are chemical. Some of these additives may prove to be helpful. BHT, a preservative to prevent staleness in bread, has been found to prolong the life of mice by as much as one-third of their normal life span. There is a possibility that some of these substances in cereals may have had an important role in dramatically decreasing the incidence of stomach cancer.

Water, fat, protein, carbohydrate, vitamins, minerals—these are what food is made of. These are the forms of the various chemicals that the body processes to provide energy for your activities and your continued health.

3

GETTING IT TO YOUR ENERGY CELLS

You will need a general concept of the circulation of food. Most people think of circulation as a means of providing oxygen to the cells and removing the carbon dioxide. This is true, but the purpose of the oxygen is to enable the food to be processed by the cells. This means the food has to be carried to the cells, too. Circulation is really a transport system, and it transports food as well as oxygen and other substances.

The process of extracting energy from your food begins with the chewing and mixing with saliva. The saliva contains amylase, an enzyme which acts on starch. Those salivary glands produce about a quart of saliva a day. Aside from its enzyme action on starches, saliva is used as a lubricant. If you ever swallowed anything while you had a completely dry mouth you would appreciate how important this is.

The lubricated bolus of food is milked down the long tubular structure called the esophagus on its route to the stomach. Inside the stomach the chemical actions that affect protein metabolism begin. The stomach has special cells that form hydrochloric acid and an enzyme substance called pepsin. In the presence of hydrochloric acid pepsin starts breaking down the complex proteins from meat, fish, milk, cereal, and other sources into smaller units. The stomach normally produces over a quart of acid pepsin juice a day. Those individuals who have an ulcer commonly produce much larger quantities of acid pepsin juice, and it contains much more hydrochloric acid as well. The only way the stomach avoids being digested itself with this powerful juice is that it is covered with a thick mucus material that protects it from the juice. When the acid juice leaks backward into the lower esophagus it can cause heartburn, or if too much squirts against the wall of the small intestine just outside the stomach, it causes a duodenal ulcer. The pepsin in our stomach has the same function as rennin in animal stomachs.

All the food you eat is churned together inside the stomach with the stomach's acid pepsin juice. Finally, the steak, apple pie, salad, and bread all become one soft uniform mixture. The stomach contracts and when part of the food is sufficiently liquid, it is squirted out of the stomach through the valvelike structure (pyloric valve) that normally closes the stomach outlet into the first part of the small intestine, the duodenum. It is important for you to realize that solid food is not readily ejected from the stomach. Solids must first be homogenized into a smooth liquid or semiliquid state. Thus, if you eat solids and lots of roughage it will be some time, usually hours, before the stomach is completely empty.

Any liquids you drink, particularly on an empty stomach, are apt to flow right through the stomach and directly into the small intestine. They don't require mixing and churning to convert them into a satisfactory state for the intestine. Of course, if the liquid is introduced into a stomach that is full of steak, salad, and bread, it is apt to be mixed into part of the solids, and its emptying time into the small intestine delayed. This is the secret of being able to drink more alcohol on a full stomach than you can on an empty one without getting drunk, at least as quickly. You still get the same amount of alcohol, but it is presented to the small intestine and, hence, the circulation at a slower rate.

It also makes a difference what kind of food you eat. If it is all carbohydrate material it will be processed rather rapidly in the stomach and emptied directly into the small intestine. It doesn't take long for bread to be mixed into a slush and emptied. Protein foods take a little longer for processing. Fats take the longest time of all, and hours after a fatty meal the stomach will still not have emptied completely. This is a major consideration when you are talking about diets and foods for problems such as low blood sugar. And it matters whether the food is hot or cold. Cold foods slow down the rhythmic contractions of the stomach and the emptying time. A cold fat solid will sit there in the stomach longest of all. If the food is warm it has the opposite effect. So it is that hot liquids tend to move directly from the stomach into the intestine and whatever they contain can be rapidly absorbed into the bloodstream.

The tearing down of whatever you have eaten and getting it ready for the bloodstream really gets down to business in the small intestine. This is where most of the action is. As the food material from the stomach (chyme) enters the duodenum it is mixed with bile from the liver, that important pancreatic juice, and the juices formed within the wall of the intestine. The latter go by a fancy name, the *succus entericus*.

There is a big job to accomplish in the intestine. The small intestine is no transparent membrane. It is considerably thicker than an inner tube for your car. The average length in an adult is twenty-two feet (about seven meters). The problem is to get the food material through this wall into the blood vessels that surround the tubelike structure and actually penetrate its wall. Unless this can be accomplished, all the food in the world is not going to help your nutrition. This is not just a simple mechanical process. There is no pump to force the chyme into the circulation, and if it did pass through in this state it would make you sick. The process has to be accomplished by various enzymes splitting the food down into some basic chemicals and then passing these fragments of what you have eaten into the circulation.

Our food doesn't just squeeze through between the cells that form the intestinal wall, either. That wall is essentially water- and air-tight. The basic chemical elements from your food must be absorbed into the cells that line the intestine, then transported to the circulation by complex chemical actions requiring energy. This is why very little of the things you eat, other than water, salts, and minerals, are likely to be found in their original chemical state within the circulation. Failure to recognize this causes many people to be misled by test-tube research. It isn't enough to see what happens to a food in a test tube and then decide that the same thing will happen if you swallow it. Your food must be chemically processed before it gets into the circulation. Even ordinary table sugar doesn't get into your circulation as table sugar dissolved in water. If you don't have the right enzymes in the intestine, you won't even be able to use it for food.

You should keep in mind that almost all of the absorption of food material occurs in the small intestine. The bile acts to emulsify or make fat particles more soluble so they can be absorbed into the cells. The pancreatic juice contains important enzymes that help to break down the carbohydrates, fats, and proteins.

Once the basic chemical nutrients have been absorbed into the cells they pass into the circulation. The amino acids from the proteins and the single sugars from carbohydrates are absorbed into the small veins that surround the small intestine. Most of the fat is picked up by the lymphatics.

What are the lymphatics? They are another circulatory system in the body that you haven't heard much about because they have nothing to do with carrying oxygen, and contain no red blood cells. There are small lymph glands all over your body. They are about the same as the tonsils, which are really very large lymph glands. They are connected by small vessels. If you have ever injured yourself and seen clear liquid material expressed, the chances are you were looking at lymph, the fluid formed by the lymph glands. If you have had a sore throat and felt those glands around the neck, you were feeling inflamed lymph glands. One of their main functions is to form the white blood cells used to defend the body against infection or even unacceptable foreign matter. This immense network of lymph vessels empties its fluid, containing the white blood cells, into one of the large veins that drains directly into the heart. Most of the fat particles are carried by the lymph vessels from the intestine to the same large vein, and in this way fat enters the circulation.

You may want to follow the diagram of the food circulation, Figure 1, as this discussion continues.

The nutrient-laden blood from the intestines flows to the liver in what is called the portal circulation. Here the liver begins to process the nutrients. The liver should be regarded as the main food-processing plant. It is the metabolic stabilizer (metabolostat) for the body. If you don't have enough glucose in your blood, it takes other nutrients and turns them into glucose. You will see later how it can act as a giant food changer. Its behavior is influenced by what you eat.

The nutrients that leave the liver after processing pass through the veins to the heart, and, just before arriving in the right side of the heart, the load of fatty particles is dumped into the bloodstream. The circulation is now fully loaded with the nutrients you have eaten and is transporting them to the cells for further processing.

The circulation will pass through the right side of the heart and on to the lungs. Nature was an efficient designer. Not only will the circulation carry the nutrients, but in the lungs it picks up the oxygen you will need to process them. At the same time it will release the excess carbon dioxide your cells formed in processing other nutrients. This, incidentally, will affect the body's chemical balance, called the acid-base balance —more about that later. The lungs also give off water and this also comes from the circulation. The processing of the various nutrients in the cells generates water. This water can be added to what you drink and that in the foods you eat to provide the total amount of water your body needs. That dry teaspoon of sugar you put in your coffee results in the formation of water when the cells process it for energy.

The oxygenated blood turns bright red and passes on with its nutrients to the left side of the heart and from there is pumped throughout the body. Some of the blood goes to the fat cells where some of the fat

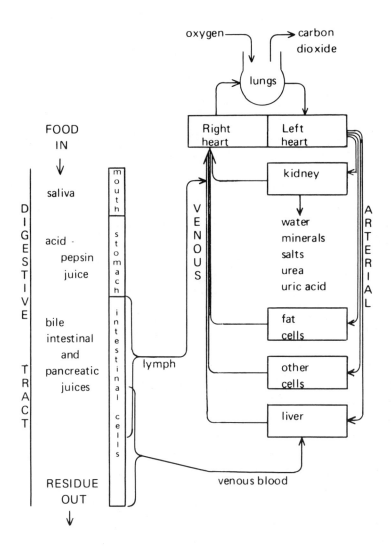

Fig. 1. Food circulation.

particles are picked up and processed. Other nutrients can also be used here to form fat. Other blood goes to muscle cells and here the nutrients are taken into the cells, processed, and converted into energy for use in muscular contractions. Still other blood goes to various glands all over the body for them to use the nutrients to form hormones, pancreatic enzymes, and other enzymes. Some will be used to produce new cells. Circulation to the blood-forming organs provides the material for those 200 million new red blood cells a minute that you need. Other nutrients are used in the lymph glands to form the white cells. And, so it is, all over the body the nutrients are used in the formation of new cells, replacement of old cells, or formation of vital body substances.

The blood that goes to the skin is of vital importance in regulating the chemistry of the body and controlling body temperature. It enables the skin to act as a giant water-evaporative cooler. You lose about a quart of water from the skin every day, even without noticeable sweating. Of course, if you sweat you lose a lot more. Its evaporation cools the surface of the body, and the cooler blood returns to cool the internal body. With loss of much sweat, salt is also lost and must be replaced from what you eat.

The circulation also carries other leftover products from the metabolic process besides carbon dioxide. These include the products left over from using the amino acids from protein, called urea, and a few other minor products. A portion of the blood loaded with oxygen and nutrients passes to the kidney. It not only provides necessary nourishment for the kidney cells, but the blood is filtered in the process. The excess salt, water, urea, and a host of other chemicals are filtered out here. Obviously, if the body needs more water, the kidney saves the water and puts out a concentrated urine. But if there is too much water accumulating, the kidney eliminates much more and dilutes other substances in the urine.

Finally, from all these various cells the circulating blood picks up the excess carbon dioxide, the excess urea, and other products, then circulates back through miles and miles of small capillaries into the veins, ready to pick up another load of nutrients from the liver and the lymph vessels, more oxygen from the lungs, and start all over again.

You should note that a part of the oxygenated blood from the arteries also goes to the liver. In this way the material released from the various body cells into their capillaries eventually gets back to the liver. If there are any toxic substances produced by the cells, it can be chemically detoxified in the liver. In addition, the fat cells can release fatty particles into the veins to circulate to the liver, where they can be processed for the body's needs.

The food left in the small intestine after the absorption process is propelled into the colon. The colon has no role in absorbing nutrients. Even though there is a large amount of vitamin B_{12} formed by bacteria living in the large colon, it can't be absorbed and used by our bodies. The main function of the colon is to absorb water and salt from the liquid slush left from the absorptive process in the small intestine. The end result is to leave a normally solid food residue of indigestible material which also contains the end products of bile, discarded cells from the intestinal tract, and products of various bacteria that normally live in the colon. Bacteria normally thrive in the colon and further break down cellulose material and nonnutrient substances.

4

YOUR ENERGY SHUTTLE

All of the carbohydrates, proteins, fats, and even alcohol we consume contain energy that is released by the metabolic action of our cells. The energy comes from the formation of chemical compounds. The chemical union of two or more elements into a compound or molecule requires energy. Tearing the molecule apart releases the energy. We know that an atom has a tremendous amount of energy stored within it. An atomic bomb releases a lot of energy because the fundamental electrical structure of the atom is broken apart, releasing the energy. On a smaller scale, when the atoms that make up a molecule are broken apart, the process releases energy.

Perhaps the best-understood example of the release of energy by the destruction of molecules is fire, to generate heat energy. When you burn coal you are tearing apart the molecules of coal, mostly carbon, and releasing energy as heat. The combustion process requires oxygen to accomplish the destruction. This is a form of metabolism. It is a distinct change induced by a chemical process called oxidation. And you can burn wood, which breaks down the cellulose material to generate heat, or burn gas or various petroleum products. A variety of chemical reactions generate energy. You can feel the heat generated in a test tube during many of these reactions.

Not all energy is in the form of heat. It can also be in the form of electricity, or light, or mechanical energy. Energy can be transformed. As you know, electrical energy can be converted into heat, light, or mechanical energy. As you will see, the energy in your food comes from the sun. In a sense we all run on solar energy.

Most of the energy used by the body is not used for either heat or physical activity. The relation of energy to heat, though, is the basis for expressing energy in calories. The calorie is a measure of heat energy. Most of the energy in the body is used for the variety of chemical actions that must take place. The energy is literally sopped up in forming new compounds, mostly protein, to replace old structures or build new ones for hormones, enzymes, and other secretions. A lot is used in the work of moving chemicals through cells, and some of the energy is dissipated as heat.

Forget the old idea that food is burned in oxygen in the cells. There are no fires in the cells. The only burning in the body is that feeling in the pit of the stomach from too much stomach acid. The body transfers energy back and forth in its chemical compounds. I sometimes call these the body's rocket fuel. You'll learn more about how these energy compounds work as we go along, but you need to develop a concept now as to how these "energy shuttles" work.

Unfortunately, all of these energy compounds have complex names, but we'll name them and then use symbols or abbreviations. These important compounds are phosphates. The one that contains the least amount of energy is called adenosine monophosphate, or AMP. In this

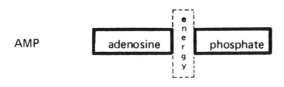

Fig. 2. The AMP (adenosine monophosphate) low-energy unit.

compound one unit of adenosine is bound to one unit of phosphate. The bond between the units holds a small amount of energy, and it can be expressed in calories. When a unit of adenosine combines with two phosphate units it is called adenosine diphosphate, or ADP. It is a much more powerful fuel and contains a great deal of energy. The additional bond to add a second phosphate group sops up a lot more energy than the single bond for AMP. The most powerful body fuel of all is a combination of one adenosine unit and three phosphate units, called adenosine triphosphate or ATP.

In the process of breaking down carbohydrates, proteins, fats, and even alcohol, their energy is used to form these high-energy compounds. Here is how the energy shuttle works. There will be some AMP in the

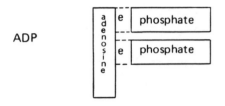

Fig. 3. The ADP (adenosine diphosphate) high-energy unit. The **e** represents energy required to bind the two
phosphate units to adenosine.

cell. As the nutrient is broken down chemically and gives up its energy, the AMP sops up the energy to bind another phosphate to it and become ADP. Or ADP sops up the energy, adds another phosphate from the chemicals in the cell, and becomes ATP. Now, when the cell needs some energy for any of its functions it takes it from the ATP. The ATP simply

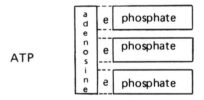

Fig. 4. The ATP (adenosine triphosphate) high-energy unit. The **e** represents the energy required to bind
three phosphate units to adenosine.

gives up its extra phosphate and the energy, converting back to ADP. Of course, ADP can release energy and phosphate and become AMP. Actually ADP and ATP are simply ways to store energy for future use.

As a result of this simple energy-shuttle mechanism the energy can be absorbed, stored (to some extent), and even transported easily throughout the body. Of course, there is some heat lost in the transaction, but it is minimal and merely represents the overhead of the transaction. You can regard the heat formed as analogous to the heat from an electric light bulb. The heat is only a secondary and unwanted product in generating light.

In addition to AMP, ADP, and ATP, the body can form a special high-energy compound found mostly in the muscles. It is called creatine phosphate, hereafter called only CP. Creatine is a protein made from three amino acids. When it is combined with phosphate to form CP it becomes

CP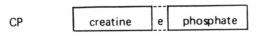

Fig. 5. The CP (creatine phosphate) high-energy unit. The e represents the energy required to bind phosphate to creatine.

a high-energy compound. It is an energy reservoir for ATP. This is how it works. As ATP is formed from the metabolic process it acts on creatine and gives it one of its phosphate energy units. The result is a unit of CP and a downgrading of ATP to ADP. The creatine really only promises to keep the phosphate energy until it is needed. During muscular contraction the energy is needed. So the ADP takes back its phosphate and energy from CP and becomes ATP again. Then the energy from ATP is used for muscular contraction.

One of the most important energy-shuttle mechanisms is a coenzyme. And just what is a coenzyme? First let's clarify what an enzyme is. There are a vast number of chemical compounds that go under this label. They are all proteins made by connecting various amino acids. Produced by living cells, their main function is to speed up or facilitate various chemical actions without being destroyed themselves. You might say they are the agitators of the chemical brawl. A coenzyme serves about the same function, but it is not a protein. Although it contains complex chemical compounds, they are not amino acids. An important coenzyme in the energy-shuttle system is called simply Coenzyme A (Co-A). It contains sulfur, which explains why some sulfur is necessary in the body. It also contains one of the vitamin-B group called pantothenic acid. (For more about this vitamin see the discussion on pantothenic acid.) Co-A combines with acetic acid to form a very active and powerful compound, active acetate. It is a cornerstone in the metabolic processing of fats, carbohydrates, proteins, and alcohol, and the formation of important compounds, including cholesterol. Yes, acetic acid is what makes vinegar vinegar. When Co-A is combined with acetic acid as active acetate it contains a lot of energy.

These, then, are the main energy shuttles your body uses: AMP, ADP, ATP, CP, and Co-A. They are the kinds of fuel storage and transfer your body uses to provide energy.

As the metabolic process continues, the broken-down parts of the food you eat must be eliminated. The process strips out the energy enclosed in the chemical bonds of the compounds of your food, and the individual chemicals freed when the bonds are broken are then eliminated. We literally rob our food of its energy and then get rid of it. Most of the chemicals we have to eliminate are simply carbon, oxygen, hydrogen, and nitrogen. This should be no surprise, since carbohydrates and fats contain only carbon, hydrogen, and oxygen. Protein merely adds nitrogen to the list.

Much, but not all, of the carbon and oxygen are eliminated as carbon dioxide, mostly through the lungs, but also some through the kidneys. As you probably know, the carbon dioxide is combined with the hemoglobin in your red blood cells and hauled to the lungs where it is released. You can think of the carbon as being eliminated by using oxygen to form carbon dioxide. This is one purpose of the oxygen you breathe. The oxygen normally in the carbohydrate molecule is also used for this purpose. Fat contains very little oxygen, and, for this reason, it takes more oxygen to eliminate the carbon from fat than it does from carbohydrates. Most of the nitrogen is converted to urea and eliminated in the urine. A small amount is eliminated as uric acid, or its salt, sodium urate.

Much of the hydrogen is also eliminated by using oxygen. The combination of hydrogen with oxygen forms ordinary water. Here again the oxygen you breathe is used to eliminate certain elements in the food you eat. The water can be used by the body just the same as the water you drink. When you talk about how much water you should drink a day, keep in mind that the body forms a lot of water from the metabolic process.

Joining the oxygen to the hydrogen produced in the cells occurs as a result of a complex chemical action. It is part of the repeated metabolic processing of your foods. If you follow the diagrams, though, a simplified version of the process isn't too difficult. The hydrogen is literally handed from one compound to another in the process, similar to the childhood game of "pass it on." The various compounds work in a bucket-brigade

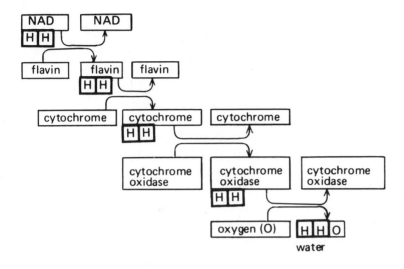

Fig. 6. How the enzyme system transports hydrogen (HH) step by step to a point where it can react with oxygen (O) to form water (HHO).

system which I sometimes call the hydrogen express. Two of the main transport mechanisms involve two more coenzymes. One of these is NAD (the chemical name is nicotinamide adeninedinucleotide). Incidentally, it contains nicotinamide or niacin, another member of the vitamin-B group. You can begin to see why vitamins are important. The normal metabolic process that gives your body energy couldn't be accomplished without them. The other coenzyme is NAD with a phosphate group added, called NADP. Both of these coenzymes have the capacity to carry two hydrogen blocks and, when they are fully loaded with hydrogen, are written as NAD.2H and NADP.2H. You can think of the end result as NAD carrying the blocks of hydrogen to a point where they can combine with oxygen to form water. Water, of course, is a unit made up of two blocks of hydrogen and one block of oxygen. The coenzymes only transport the hydrogen temporarily, and when they "pass it on" eventually to oxygen, they return to their natural state, ready to carry the next load of hydrogen.

The hydrogen blocks begin their journey carried by NAD, the niacin-containing coenzyme. They change carriers and board the flavin molecule. This is a yellow pigment compound that contains vitamin B_2, also known as riboflavin. From here they journey on to cytochrome, an iron-containing protein similar to hemoglobin. The cytochrome passes them on to cytochrome oxidase, an enzyme. The cytochrome oxidase enzyme interacts with the oxygen from respiration to pass on the hydrogen to the oxygen. This is the end of the line, with the formation of water and a return of the enzyme to its original state. As you can see from this journey, as each carrier passes on the hydrogen it returns to its original state, ready to transport another load of hydrogen.

Hydrogen can also be eliminated through the kidneys. Any nitrogen in your food that you don't need will be converted into urea and eliminated in the urine. The excess water, created by means of the hydrogen express, can also be eliminated in urine. Some of the water combines with carbon dioxide to form carbonic acid. When it gets to the lungs it is converted back to carbon dioxide and water and exhaled.

The hydrogen-express mechanism liberates energy. For each molecule of NAD that is freed from its combination with hydrogen three molecules of ATP are formed. Now get this, the formation of the ATP can be blocked and the energy converted to heat. This is what some antibiotics and thyroid hormones do. In this way thyroid hormone causes energy from food that should be used for other body functions to be converted into heat instead of ATP. As a result, the person with an overactive thyroid is hot and gets less usable energy from his food.

You can see from the way your food is handled why the doctor measures the amount of oxygen you use to evaluate your metabolism. The purpose of the oxygen is to transport the carbon and the hydrogen out of your body. By measuring the amount of oxygen you use for this purpose, he has a pretty good idea how much of your food is being converted to energy by the metabolic process.

Now that you have a general concept of how the energy is released from your food it is a good time to talk again about how the energy is used. A small amount of the energy is used for body heat. If your body temperature begins to fall, energy can be released from ATP or ADP to generate heat. But despite the fact that calories are a measure of heat, this represents only a small amount of the usage of your food calories.

Depending upon how physically active you are, more or less of the food energy is converted to mechanical energy. This is accomplished by the muscles in the body. Remember, there are also muscles in the digestive tract and the heart, as well as those you use in physical activity. The way the work of the muscle is accomplished is not completely known. We do know that the process is dependent on two proteins within the muscle fibers: actin and myosin. They are layered over each other within the muscle like a stack of sliding-door panels. When your muscles contract the panels slide over each other, shortening the muscle fiber. As your muscles relax, they slide apart. The details of how the sliding is accomplished is the unknown element. Obviously as the muscle shortens it moves whatever it is attached to, for example your finger, forearm, or leg, or in the digestive tract it squeezes down. The energy that enables the actin and myosin to slide over each other is supplied by ATP being converted to ADP. I mentioned earlier that ATP is replenished by the stores of CP. Both of these substances, though, could be exhausted in a very short time. The metabolic process of tearing down foods yields the energy for continuously forming more ATP to keep the action going.

For most of us, the majority of our energy is used in the building and transporting processes in our body. Let's take another look at how the energy is used to build those active bodies of young children or to replace our worn-out cells. Each cell contains an assembly plant called the ribosomes. Inside the ribosome is the vital nucleic acid, RNA. The RNA, too, is built from chemicals that come from your food. You can think of the strip of RNA as a string of bolts tied together by their heads. The free end of each bolt can be fitted with a nut of the right size. These nuts are the various amino acids. Obviously only the right-sized nut will fit the right bolt. The same thing is true with RNA and the amino acids—only the right amino acid will fit at a point on the RNA chain. By a complex mechanism, the amino acids are all lined up at the right spot along the strand of RNA.

You could hook all the nuts to the bolts together, but it would require energy, by welding them together. The amino acids are all hooked together and it takes energy; but rather than heat, it is a chemical action, and the energy is taken from the ATP. The chain of amino acids is the body protein. You can manufacture any number of proteins using different amino acids or hooking them together in different sequences—just like making words out of the alphabet. Actually the entire process of making our body proteins uses only about twenty-one amino acids, fewer building blocks for all those complex proteins than there are letters in the alphabet. It's enough, though. Just think how many words in different languages you can make with only twenty-six building blocks.

The amino acids used for building blocks come from your food and so does the energy to hook them together. As the process continues, then, your food becomes your body, so you are what you eat.

5

WHAT ARE CARBOHYDRATES?

If you are confused about all those different terms used for carbohydrates, join the club. The list is pretty formidable and includes starch (and that can be animal or vegetable), sugar, glucose, lactose, maltose, dextrose, sucrose, levulose, fructose, galactose, dextrin, glycogen, invert sugar, monosaccharides, disaccharides, and polysaccharides. You can add to this list hexose, pentose, pectins, and cellulose. Yet, despite all those names, the whole thing is pretty simple.

To begin with, carbohydrates are compounds of carbon, hydrogen, and oxygen. They get their name from the idea that they are hydrates of carbon (watered carbon) and indeed they are. It is a bit difficult to realize that water combined with the carbon you see in charcoal is that sweet sugar you use, but that's the wonderful thing about how Nature arranges things.

The formation of carbohydrates is a good illustration of the interdependence of the animal and vegetable kingdom and a wonderful example of how energy can be converted. The process begins with the energy from the sun. The green plants all around us contain chlorophyll. It takes the carbon dioxide out of the air, combines it with the hydrogen from water, and, using the energy from the sun, binds it all together as carbohydrate. In the process, oxygen from the water is freed and emitted into the atmosphere. The plant provides life-giving oxygen for us at the same time it is manufacturing carbohydrates for our food. The sun's energy is converted into chemical energy and eventually will end up in the ATP molecules in your body. So, in the last analysis, our bodies are run by the energy of the sun.

The simplest unit of carbohydrates is a monosaccharide or single sugar. It can't be broken down into any smaller unit except by chemical actions such as occur in the metabolic process. You can think of it as being built from six units of water and six blocks of carbon. The way these can be arranged can be relatively complex, but it is just as easy to think of a monosaccharide as a set of blocks placed together. Any child who can use a Tinker Toy set or build with blocks can do it. Here is a block diagram of a monosaccharide. By a minor rearrangement of the block formation you can produce the three important monosaccharides. Because each monosaccharide contains six carbon atoms it is often called a hexose.

The three important monosaccharides are glucose, fructose, and galactose. Of these, glucose is by far the most important to us. All carbohydrates

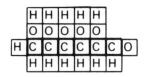

Fig. 7. A simplified block diagram of a monosaccharide, such as ordinary glucose.

are converted to this form to be used by the cells for energy. Both fructose and galactose are converted to glucose in the body before they are processed. Glucose and dextrose (d-glucose) are essentially the same thing. Glucose is found in fruit, milk, and starch from any source. Fructose is also called levulose. Galactose has only one name, thank goodness.

By combining two single sugars (monosaccharides), a double sugar (disaccharide) is formed. This is the form of carbohydrate most familiar to you. Ordinary table sugar is simply a combination of glucose and fructose (or by other names, dextrose and levulose). It will dissolve in water all right, but you will not be able to use much of it unless you have a special enzyme system in your intestine—which most of us have. Another double sugar is maltose, a combination of two units of glucose. The third common double sugar is lactose, the sugar in milk, produced by lactating. It is a combination of galactose and glucose. Sucrose, maltose, and galactose are the three important double sugars. When you hear someone talking about invert sugar, what they mean is a sugar of equal amounts of glucose and fructose.

It is important to understand the nature of the sugars if you want to avoid misinformation. As a case in point, Adelle Davis wrote, in *Let's Eat*

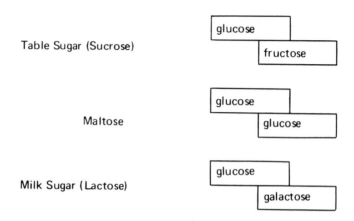

Fig. 8. How the only three important double sugars are formed from the only three important single sugars.

Right to Keep Fit, "The most valuable sugar is lactose, which occurs only in milk. It digests less readily than other sugars and apparently sometimes not at all; for this reason lactose is not fattening." Such a statement has no relation to reality. As I pointed out, lactose is a double sugar of glucose and galactose. The galactose is converted to glucose in the liver. The glucose from lactose is every bit as fattening and contains just as much energy as the glucose in table sugar or corn syrup. Glucose is glucose. Having been raised on the farm myself, I was astonished that Adelle Davis's frequently reported Indiana farm experience failed to impress her with the value of skim milk to fatten pigs and young calves. Some adults do have trouble absorbing lactose because they can't split the double sugar (more on that later), and milk makes these people sick with indigestion.

If you join more than two units of single sugars it is called a polysaccharide or poly sugar. Starch, cellulose, and pectin are all examples of a poly sugar. The human digestive tract cannot digest either cellulose or pectins, so our interest here is in the starch. The formation of double sugars is achieved by eliminating one unit of water from the two single sugars at the one point where the blocks of carbon from each sugar are joined. The process is simply repeated to form long chains of sugar units or starch. The plants make starch entirely from glucose, and when it is broken down for use, it is a source of glucose. Cornstarch, for example,

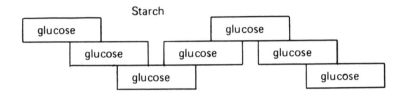

Fig. 9. How glucose units are used to build starch.

can be converted to pure glucose by adding water and subjecting it to a chemical process that breaks it apart. The product, corn syrup, is a good source of pure glucose (dextrose). It is a concentrated solution of a single sugar, glucose.

The starch granules are stored in the roots and seeds of plants. Potatoes are an excellent example of a plant's storehouse for starch. Corn is a good example of its storage in seeds, as are all the cereals. Animals store starch also, and the animal starch is called glycogen. This is an important compound for you to remember. It is also formed by combining multiple units of glucose. In a sense it is concentrated glucose since, in its formation, some water is removed. Glycogen is the immediate source of energy for the body when you are without food for any reason. It is stored in the liver as a ready source of energy for the body as a whole and in the muscles as an immediate source of energy for muscular activity.

Cellulose also is a combination of the carbon blocks of the units of glucose. The big difference is that the carbon blocks are joined at several locations. We are unable to break down these multiple bonds. The plant-eating animals are, and many of them use cellulose for energy. The multiple bonds used in forming cellulose make it much stronger. This greater strength is the way plant fibers that constitute the skeleton of the plant are formed. The cellulose sometimes surrounds starch granules making it impossible for man to digest the raw starch. Cooking plant starch breaks down starch granules and removes the cellulose case that may be present. This makes it possible for the various enzymes in the body to break down starch into glucose so it can be used by the body.

Some other carbohydrates are relatively unimportant as far as food energy is concerned. Some of these are quite important to cell function, such as the pentoses, whose name means there are only five carbon blocks in the formation. They are among the nucleic acids in the cell

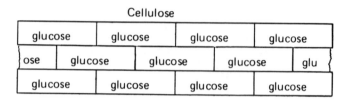

Fig. 10. How glucose units are used to build cellulose.

nucleus, and we will have more to say about them later. Carbohydrates can be combined with fats and proteins to make more complex compounds needed for the body's structure.

Honey and corn syrup are common foods containing only single sugars. Honey is a mixture of the single sugars glucose and fructose. They are not connected as a double sugar. Corn syrup is only glucose. There is no advantage in eating honey over corn syrup or sugar, for that matter, unless you have a problem absorbing double sugars from your intestine. Besides, the fructose in honey is rapidly converted to glucose.

How much carbohydrate do you need in your diet each day? There is no definite answer to that. It depends on how many calories you need and what else you are eating. It seems that you will need at least 50 grams or about 200 calories from carbohydrates every day at a minimum, if you don't want to upset your body chemistry. You will learn more about that in the discussion of low-carbohydrate fad diets. The body needs enough calories each day to provide energy for the constant chemical changes that occur in the body, the transportation problem, the new-cells-for-old bit, as well as formation of vital secretions, and for your daily activity.

Keep in mind it is energy you need, and carbohydrates, protein, fat, and alcohol all contain energy which we measure as calories. It is much like having money from several different countries. If you are going to spend some to add to your wardrobe it really doesn't matter whether it is German marks, French francs, or American dollars. You can exchange them back and forth and use their buying energy to make your purchases. If you have very little fat in your diet you will need more carbohydrates to increase the available energy for your cells. You can also use proteins for energy by breaking them down into their chemical blocks and robbing them of their energy. The only reason not to is that you need an adequate amount of the amino acids in the proteins to use as building blocks for the cells and their many protein products. By eating carbohydrates and fats we spare the amino acids in proteins from being torn down to provide energy.

Does it make any difference how your carbohydrates are packaged, that is, whether it is as sugar, starch, milk, or whole vegetables and cereals? Yes, it does. I think this is one of the most important points about carbohydrates and one that is commonly missed. It's true that starch, honey, syrups, carbohydrates in fruit, vegetables, berries, and cereals all end up as glucose. The difference is in the speed with which the conversion is accomplished. If the food takes a glucose express highway to the bloodstream, the amount of glucose in your blood will rise rapidly after you have eaten it. If, on the other hand, it takes time to process the carbohydrate it will be a while before the blood-glucose level rises. Even then, because the effect is spread out, the high peak levels may not occur. (Incidentally, the correct term is blood glucose, although blood sugar is commonly used.) The key to how fast a carbohydrate enters the bloodstream is mostly related to how the stomach processes food. You can see how packaging effects this by tracing the processing of some common foods that are mostly carbohydrate.

The effects of how the carbohydrate is packaged start in the mouth. Let's assume you are going to eat a bowl of shredded wheat with milk and sugar. Of these three foods, only sugar is just carbohydrate. Most foods in their natural state are a mixture of protein, fat, and carbohydrate. Table sugar, sucrose, is a double sugar or disaccharide composed entirely of glucose and fructose. Shredded wheat is 75 per cent carbohydrate in the form of starch. That means tightly packaged glucose units hooked together. Some cellulose as cereal fiber adds to its bulk, but we can't digest it. The bulk is very important because it aids in the normal function of the colon. If you use whole milk, about one-third of its calories will be carbohydrate, less than a fourth will be protein, and nearly half its calories will be fat. If you use skim milk, fortified with nonfat milk solids, a greater percentage of its calories will be protein. A little more than half its calories will be carbohydrate and a little less than half will be from protein. The carbohydrate in milk is lactose, a double sugar composed of galactose and glucose.

As soon as you start chewing, things begin to happen to this package. The saliva contains amylase, sometimes called ptyalin, an enzyme that breaks down starch. It will start breaking down the starch in the shredded wheat into smaller units and finally into maltose. Remember, maltose is a double sugar made up of two units of glucose. The saliva will have no effect on any of the other foods in your bowl of cereal. How long the amylase will act on your shredded wheat depends on how well you chew it. The chemical environment can't be too acid or it will destroy its action. By chewing and chewing it will have time to act on a lot of the starch, but if it is swallowed immediately the acid in the stomach may stop this activity. If the just-swallowed shredded wheat is in the center of a food bolus, protected somewhat from the acid juices swirling around on the outside of the mass of more solid food, then the activity can continue a bit longer.

You may have heard that raw starch cannot be digested. That is partially true. You need to cook starch to break it down into smaller units that can interact more easily with amylase. Many of these smaller units are properly called dextrin. Shredded wheat is cooked in its preparation, and this makes it easier to digest than a raw potato.

Once the shredded wheat, sugar, and milk arrive in the stomach, they are churned mightily. In the process, they are mixed with any other food you might have in your stomach. None of it is allowed to be squirted out of the stomach until it is in a liquid or near-liquid form. Liquids pass quickly through the stomach. Emptying the stomach depends on a host of factors, but, as a guide, ordinary water passes through the stomach directly into the small intestine almost as fast as you can swallow it. The liquids in your diet spread out over the surface of the stomach, surrounding the solid-food bolus being worked upon. The liquid part of your diet that isn't absorbed into the food bolus then moves very rapidly into the small intestine. If you use a lot of milk on your shredded wheat or drink other liquids, or if there is enough fluid in the stomach, you can expect a reasonable portion of the milk and the dissolved sugar to pass directly into the small intestine. There won't be much of the fluid or any food material absorbed from the stomach into the circulation. Less than 3 per cent of water is absorbed per minute from the stomach, while over 25 per cent of the water you drink is absorbed in a minute from the small intestine.

The shredded wheat is kept in the stomach to be churned, then gradually emptied into the small intestine. This is not true of the milk and sugar. As the food arrives in the small intestine the acid stomach juice is neutralized and the digestive juices from the pancreas, intestinal wall, and bile encounter the food. The pancreatic juice contains more amylase and it goes to work on the starch granules from the shredded wheat, when they finally arrive. It splits them down to the double-sugar maltose, composed of two units of glucose. The amylase isn't necessary to process the table sugar and milk sugar since these are already in the form of double sugars.

The double sugars cannot be absorbed directly into the cells of the intestinal lining. There is some controversy about where the action takes place, whether in the juices from the intestinal wall or within the cells that line the small intestine. In either case, you must have an enzyme to split the double sugars into single sugars. The enzyme that splits table sugar (sucrose) into glucose and fructose is sucrase. Maltase splits the maltose from the shredded wheat into two units of glucose, and the lactase splits the lactose in the milk into galactose and glucose. Now they are ready to be processed through the rest of the intestinal wall and finally picked up in the bloodstream. Note, all that is left of the food is three single sugars, the only ones important to food energy: glucose, fructose, and galactose. This is the fate of all carbohydrates in the form of usable food.

The level of glucose in the blood (blood sugar) will be affected by the absorption of these foods into the bloodstream. All of the single sugars are carried by the bloodstream to the liver. Here galactose is converted to glucose and part of the fructose is converted to glucose. The rest of the fructose is converted to glucose in the muscles before it can be processed to strip it of its energy.

Only a very small amount of the sugars can be absorbed from the intestine by simple diffusion across the wall of the intestine. They must be transported chemically. The glucose in the intestine, and other single sugars, will move across the intestinal wall into the blood even when there is more glucose in the blood than in the food solution inside the intestine. Thus, the movement across the wall is not accomplished simply because there is more glucose inside the intestine than there is in the blood. As the concentration of the sugars in the food solution is increased, up to a point, the absorption will be more rapid. The rate of absorption is not increased further when the concentration of the sugars in the intestine exceeds the concentration of sugars in the blood. Instead, the rate of absorption remains the same. The actual movement of the sugars through the intestinal-wall cells requires energy, and this is supplied by our chemical energy source, ATP. Within the intestinal cells the ATP breaks down to ADP and the energy is used up in transporting the sugars across the intestinal wall into the bloodstream. The sugars are all absorbed within the first three feet of the small intestine.

Obviously, as the single sugars are absorbed into the bloodstream, they will cause the blood-glucose level to rise. The degree of the rise will depend on how much sugar is absorbed. That is a very important principle because it has a lot to do with such problems as low blood sugar and even your sensation of hunger.

The shredded wheat is emptied slowly from the stomach into the intestine so its starch–to maltose–to glucose process takes quite a bit longer, and the material is gradually made available to the small intestine for absorption. As a result, a carbohydrate like shredded wheat cannot cause a sharp rise in the blood-glucose level. By contrast, the sugar and milk will move rapidly into the small intestine and tend to cause a more rapid rise in the blood-glucose level. For this reason sweet liquids are more likely to cause a sharp increase in blood glucose than solids, particularly those solids that contain bulk. You can see that a cup of hot, sweet coffee will cause a peak rise in the blood glucose. You would never experience this from shredded wheat alone, or from the many vegetables that contain moderate or small amounts of carbohydrate locked in with roughage, bulk, or indigestible material. You can also understand why the doctor gives the diabetic who has had too much insulin and gone into an insulin shock a glass of orange juice with sugar in it. The sweet juice goes directly into the small intestine without delay in the stomach and provides quick relief from the symptoms of low blood glucose.

Most of the bulky vegetables will delay emptying of the stomach and smooth out the absorption of sugars into the blood. You can include in this group broccoli, cabbage, and other leafy vegetables; many of the root vegetables, such as radishes; and many of the whole cereals. The plain starches like those in boiled potatoes and peas take longer for processing in the stomach than any liquid nourishment, but not as long as the more bulky foods.

There is considerable variation in how the fruit and berry group will be processed. All of the juices will normally move rapidly through the stomach and will increase the blood glucose rapidly. So will the juices that run out of the oranges, grapefruit, and similar fruits. When the starch and sugars are encased in a more fibrous material, as in a fresh apple, it will take the stomach longer to convert this to a liquid material and, hence, delay its absorption and effects on the blood-glucose level.

A food like pancakes will be easily dissolved in the stomach and will be emptied into the intestine fairly quickly. It will help run the blood-glucose level up. The same applies to many of the bread-group foods, particularly those made with refined flour devoid of cereal fiber.

Most cakes and desserts behave in a similar fashion and, of course, have a longer-lasting effect because of the large amount of sugar in them.

You might think ice cream would act this way too. The fact is that ice cream may slow down the emptying process of the stomach. Why? Because it is cold. The cold solution will slow down the stomach contractions and it may be some time before it is emptied into the intestine. And ice cream usually contains a lot of fat, which takes longer for processing within the stomach.

You might ask if using honey will decrease the speed of the rise in the blood glucose. No, it won't. The only advantage to honey, other than its flavor, is that it is made up of single sugars, glucose and fructose, and does not contain any double sugars. For this reason, people who cannot tolerate table sugar, because they lack the enzyme sucrase needed to split it into glucose and fructose for absorption, may tolerate honey.

A word needs to be said about the importance of the enzymes in the intestine which split the common double sugars. Many adults do not have any lactase, the enzyme needed to split the milk sugar lactose into galactose and glucose. These people cannot tolerate milk or milk products. The unabsorbed milk sugar acts somewhat like a chemical laxative. It can cause lots of gas, distention, abdominal cramping, and real misery. The problem was not generally recognized until recent years. Since you can't see it on an x-ray or in many laboratory tests, people who had "indigestion" on this basis were often considered "nervous" at best and sometimes "crocks" by the medical profession. Now we know a lot more about this problem and recognize how common it is. Only the people who are of Northern-European descent can usually tolerate much milk as adults. Most of the other peoples of the world have a limited tolerance to lactose. This includes Africans, Asians, American Indians, and the Mediterranean people.

Intolerance to lactose is not usually absolute. Many of these people can use some lactose without getting sick, but when they begin to use more trouble begins. Much of the adult world is spared this problem because there isn't that much milk available for use in food, but in the milk-drinking countries this problem is often seen. It is also seen rather frequently in adults of Northern-European extraction. Some people with lactose intolerance can tolerate milk products made from the fermentation process or souring, such as cheese, yogurt, and buttermilk. The lactose content will be sufficiently lowered to be within their tolerance. This may be one reason why some people use buttermilk rather than plain milk.

A similar problem can occur for the other two double sugars, maltose and sucrose, if their enzymes, maltase and sucrase, are absent. You can lose these enzymes temporarily rather than as an inherited trait, for example, during an illness that affects the lining of the small intestine. For this reason, during some diarrhealike problems the best approach is to eliminate all the sources of double sugars until the acute condition is over and the intestinal lining has had a chance to heal.

6

GETTING ENERGY FROM CARBOHYDRATES

All the carbohydrate foods you eat are eventually converted to one single chemical compound, glucose. It contains only six carbon blocks and six units of water (twelve hydrogen blocks and six oxygen blocks). As glucose, all carbohydrates are either processed for storage or stripped of their energy from the sun used to bind their chemical blocks together. The separated blocks are discarded. The first steps of the chemical process to break glucose down into its individual chemical blocks are unique to glucose, but the later steps in the chemical process to release energy are exactly the same for glucose, proteins, fats, and alcohol. What's more, a large part of the process is reversible. This means that you can rebuild glucose or you can use some amino acids and a small part of fat (glycerol) to manufacture glucose. By using these mechanisms it is possible for the body to keep the level of blood glucose in a relatively narrow range—regardless of what you eat, if your digestion is normal.

It's important to remember that the amount of glucose in the blood is important only in relation to providing glucose in the cells. It really makes no difference what the blood glucose (sugar) is but rather what the concentration of glucose within the body cells is. Nothing happens in the bloodstream to provide energy for your body. The action is inside the cell, and it is accomplished by the tiny mitochondria system, which is nothing more or less than a processing line to disconnect the various chemical building blocks of food, releasing the energy to the AMP, ADP, ATP energy system.

Just as you provide energy to strike a match to light a fire, the processing of glucose is started by energizing it. This is done simply by adding one unit of phosphate, with its energy, to the glucose unit. The result is glucose phosphate. This is accomplished by ATP releasing one unit of phosphate energy to become ADP. The glucose phosphate can then be converted to glycogen, animal starch. Glycogen is formed by connecting hundreds of glucose units. It is stored in two places in the body, the liver and muscles. It is a basic energy reserve, or tank of fuel, for the body.

When you don't eat for any reason the liver glycogen is simply broken down and converted to glucose phosphate and made available for energy. It can also be converted to simple blood glucose to stabilize and maintain

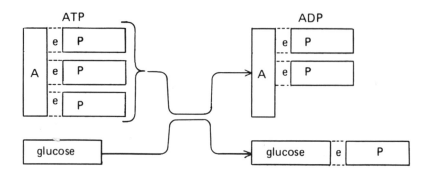

Fig. 11. The use of energy in ATP to form glucose phosphate.

your blood-glucose level. This is exactly what happens those first two days when a person goes on a starvation diet or one of the fad low-carbohydrate or no-carbohydrate diets. In all, there are about 3½ ounces of glycogen in the liver that can be used for this purpose. This provides about 400 calories, or the minimal amount of carbohydrates the body needs for two days. Remember that it takes 200 calories of carbohydrates, or about 50 grams, a day to keep your body chemistry in balance. After this initial two-day period your body chemistry becomes unbalanced, and in starvation or no-carbohydrate intake you will develop a condition called ketosis. You will understand this better after you have read about the metabolics of fat.

The muscle glycogen cannot be so easily converted back to blood glucose. It can't be readily circulated to other cells in the body to serve their needs. It is mostly trapped in the muscle. It is converted, when needed, to glucose phosphate within the muscle cell and then processed to provide energy for muscular work. A person's blood glucose can be so low it causes him to go into shock and die while his muscle cells retain most of their glycogen. Although many cells in the body can use fat for their energy source, some brain and nerve cells need glucose, apparently being unable to strip fat of its energy and use it for their cell function. This is why the brain is particularly sensitive to low blood-glucose levels. When the blood level falls there is not enough glucose in the brain cells and not enough energy for the brain cells to function normally. It is like trying to use a light bulb without any electrical energy.

Within the cells the six-carbon unit of glucose phosphate receives one more unit of energy phosphate from ATP and, through a series of reactions, divides into two units of phosphoglyceraldehyde. (I know that's a difficult word but surely not impossible to a generation Walt Disney taught to sing Mary Poppins' "Supercalifragilisticexpialidocious.") To keep things simple, I'll abbreviate it to PGA. Just think of it as the six-carbon glucose phosphate chain broken into two pieces. Each unit contains only three carbon blocks, and its own phosphate, and energy stolen from ATP. The glyceraldehyde refers to the basic three-carbon unit, and the term comes from glycerin, the oily substance used for hand lotions and innumerable compounds. Glycerin is a part of the fat particles. You will see how glycerin is processed in the discussion of using fat.

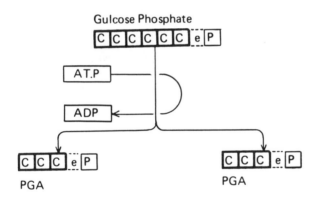

Fig. 12. The use of ATP energy to form PGA (phosphoglyceraldehyde) by splitting the simple glucose chain in half.

Once the six-carbon glucose unit has been changed into two units of three-carbon chains it is ready to yield energy. By a series of complex chemical actions it is converted to pyruvic acid. During this conversion the basic three-carbon blocks stick together. Some of the hydrogen blocks are stripped off and transported by the "hydrogen express" to the point where they can unite with oxygen within the cell to form water. This is where NAD, the hydrogen-carrying coenzyme, functions in the process. As you recall, NAD contains niacin (nicotinamide), so this is one place where niacin is necessary in processing glucose. As two blocks of hydrogen are stripped from the three-carbon skeleton and united with oxygen to form water, enough energy is released to form three units of ATP. This process, called aerobic metabolism, requires oxygen. In the process of rearranging the blocks to form pyruvic acid, enough energy is released to form two more units of ATP. Since the six-carbon chain of glucose provides two of the three-carbon chain units, there is enough energy to form a total of ten units of ATP. It took two units of energy to activate the glucose to begin the process, so there is a net release of enough energy to form eight units of ATP through this process.

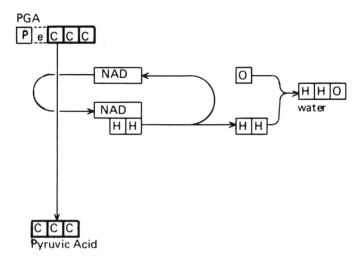

Fig. 13. The enzyme system is used to remove hydrogen (HH) from PGA to form pyruvic acid.

The entire process I've described so far of the production of pyruvic acid is reversible in each of its steps to the point of producing glucose. The glucose can be released back into the bloodstream. There is only one more important reversible step in the metabolic process for glucose. One three-carbon unit of pyruvic acid can take on a unit of carbon dioxide to form an important four-carbon unit, oxaloacetic acid. Let's abbreviate that to OAA. It takes energy to form the additional bonds between the blocks of the carbon-dioxide unit and the blocks of the pyruvic-acid unit. The process is reversible, yielding carbon dioxide, energy, and pyruvic acid. The four-carbon unit is essential to the processing of the rest of the pyruvic acid to its end point and for processing fatty acids or the carbon skeletons of amino acids from proteins.

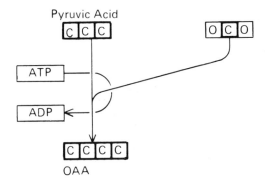

Fig. 14. The energy from ATP is used to form OAA (oxaloacetic acid) from carbon dioxide (OCO) and pyruvic acid.

The unit of pyruvic acid slated for complete processing first gives up a unit of carbon dioxide with its energy bond. The carbon dioxide and the energy unit can be used to form the four-carbon chain oxaloacetic acid from the other unit of pyruvic acid. This process also uses the hydrogen carrier NAD again, yielding more energy for ATP. It also uses the other energy shuttle vehicle, Co-A. The Co-A combines with the leftover two-carbon chain from the pyruvic acid to form active acetate. You will recall that active acetate is the combination of Co-A and acetic acid, the substance that makes vinegar.

The breakdown of pyruvic acid to active acetate is an irreversible step. The pyruvic acid is now on its way through the common metabolic grinder that strips most of the energy from the foods you eat and leaves them as disconnected blocks of carbon dioxide and water. The process is known as the citric-acid cycle or Krebs cycle, after the man who first described it. It is the common "energy circle" that releases energy from

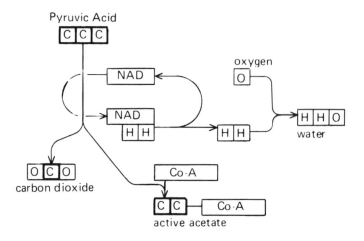

Fig. 15. The use of the hydrogen express enzyme system to convert pyruvic acid to active acetate.

glucose, fatty acids, amino acids, and alcohol. The four-carbon chain OAA combines with the active acetate to yield citric acid with a six-carbon chain skeleton. The energy used to accomplish the binding comes from splitting off Co-A which is then free to start its cycle again.

You can think of the four-carbon chain OAA as the carrier for the two-carbon fragment of acetic acid. In a series of actions two carbon blocks are stripped from the citric-acid chain, combined with oxygen, and left as units of carbon dioxide. The leftover product is a four-carbon unit of OAA which is ready to make the cycle again. It carries unit after unit of acetic acid to the grinder to be disconnected and stripped of its energy. Or the OAA can be converted back to pyruvic acid and end up as blood glucose.

The entire process of breaking pyruvic acid down to carbon dioxide, water, and energy requires oxygen. The combination of OAA with acetic acid for these actions is exactly the same for fats, proteins, and alcohol when they are used for energy. The breakdown of one unit of six-carbon glucose (two units of pyruvic acid) in its entirety from glucose to carbon dioxide yields enough energy to form thirty-eight units of ATP. The energy stored in the ATP energy shuttle can then be used to form new

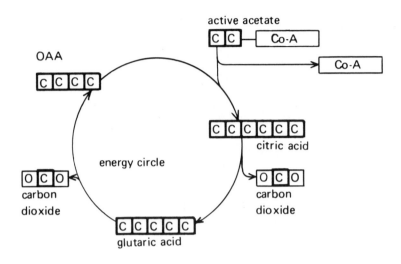

Fig. 16. The energy circle (citric-acid cycle).

cells; form enzymes, hormones, and other secretions; move chemicals across cells; accomplish mechanical work, or perform any of the other remarkable functions of the body.

Now that you have seen each stage of the processing line to disconnect glucose, you can look at the entire scheme. Read the flow diagram just as you would a map. Follow the arrows. The direction of the arrows indicates the possible paths that can be taken. When there are two arrows between two locations on the map, it is a two-way street or a reversible process. As an example, pyruvic acid to OAA is reversible. You can go from OAA to pyruvic acid, or from pyruvic acid to OAA. The process from pyruvic acid to active acetate is a one-way street with no return, so only one arrow is indicated on the flow diagram.

You can see that most of the process is reversible, except the pyruvic acid to active acetate route and the pathway around the energy circle. This is an important concept, as you will see better later.

Some amino acids from proteins can use those reversible pathways to become glucose. Some of them can't because they have been converted to acetic acid, and there is no pathway to take to become glucose for these amino acids. So only by using the proper streets can you get from some amino acids to blood glucose. By the same token, the glycerol from fat is changed into glucose by using reversible pathways. Study this simple diagram well and you will understand easily how the fats, protein, and alcohol all fit into the pathway used for glucose.

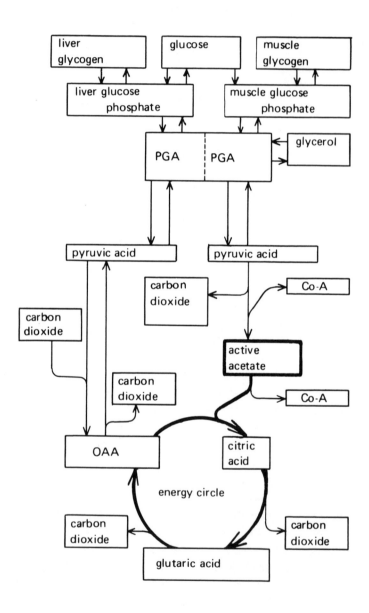

Fig. 17. The main steps in glucose metabolics.

7

WHAT ARE FATS?

You may be getting over half your calories from fat. This is a distinct departure from man's earlier history. In most instances man originally got over half of his calories from vegetables and vegetable products—cereals, fruit, berries, and other foods that are mostly carbohydrates. Many scientists, including most heart specialists, believe that the increase in fat in the diet has a lot to do with heart and vascular disease. The Inter-Society Commission on Heart Disease sponsored by the National Institutes of Health and the American Heart Association recommended that not more than 35 per cent of the calories in the diet should be from fat. Fat foods are usually the highest-calorie foods. One gram of fat contains nine calories, more than twice as many calories as you find in either proteins or carbohydrates. With the new labeling laws on food you'll need to know the differences in fats and what it all means.

Fat is made up of glycerol connected to fatty acids. Glycerol is another name for glycerin, often used in hand lotions. It is a three-carbon chain combined with three units of water and two additional blocks of hydrogen. Figure 18 will show you how the blocks are put together. As you see, it looks a lot like a carbohydrate and in the metabolic scheme of things it behaves as a carbohydrate. Technically it is an alcohol, and if it had one less carbon block with a few other changes it would be drinking alcohol. And it does contain calories.

The fatty acids all have carbon skeletons. Unlike carbohydrates they don't contain so many oxygen building blocks. You can visualize the form of a fatty acid from this diagram. It is a chain of carbon blocks joined in a single row. Different fatty acids have different numbers of carbon blocks. On each side of the carbon chain is a hydrogen block. At one end of the carbon chain there are two blocks of oxygen. You need more oxygen to get the energy out of fat than you do to use carbohy-

Fig. 18. How carbon (C), hydrogen (H), and oxygen (O) are used to form glycerol.

drates. That's because there are so few oxygen building blocks in the fatty acid.

Are you confused by the terms monoglyceride, diglyceride, and triglyceride on the ingredient labels of your food? Fatty acids can be bound to glycerol by eliminating ordinary water. If you combine only one fatty acid with glycerol, it is a monoglyceride. If you combine two fatty acids

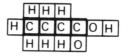

Fig. 19. A simplified block diagram of a fatty acid.

with glycerol, it is a diglyceride, and if you attach three fatty acids to glycerol it is a triglyceride. You can visualize the triglyceride unit then as three fatty acids and one glycerol unit.

The measurement of triglycerides in the blood is now a fairly common examination by many doctors. It is simply a measurement of the units of fat existing as three fatty acids bound to one glycerol unit. It is generally believed to be of use in evaluating a person's tendency to develop fatty particles in the blood vessels, called atherosclerosis, leading to heart disease and strokes.

Those discussions you have heard about saturated fat and unsaturated fat apply to the fatty acids. It is important that you understand the differences among the various fats if you are going to be able to follow the recommendations concerning your food. The classification is based on the number of hydrogen blocks the fatty acid contains. A saturated fat has two hydrogen blocks attached to each carbon block, except at the end of the chain where the oxygen is located. There is no room for any more hydrogen blocks to be attached to the carbon skeleton. Unsaturated fatty acids have one or more locations where hydrogen blocks are missing. Because of the characteristics of the carbon blocks, if any hydrogen

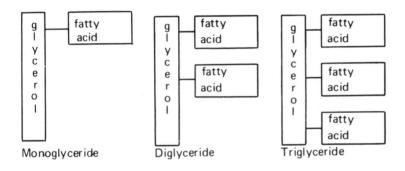

Fig. 20. How fatty acids and glycerol are used to form the common fats, mono-, di-, and triglycerides.

blocks are missing there will be a pair of carbon blocks side by side, with a missing hydrogen block. So the hydrogen blocks are missing in pairs.

When one pair of hydrogen blocks is missing from two carbon blocks, the fatty acid is called a monounsaturated fatty acid. If there are two or more spots on the carbon skeleton where pairs of hydrogen blocks are missing, it is called a polyunsaturated fatty acid.

Most heart specialists believe you should not only limit the total amount of fat in your diet but particularly the amount of calories from saturated fat. There is also some evidence that you should have about as much polyunsaturated fat in your diet as saturated fat. This is based on several decades of world-wide studies and many animal and laboratory studies. Very little is said about monounsaturated fat. It is not considered either good or bad, other than its contribution to the total fat intake and the calories they add to the diet.

A triglyceride is usually made up of three different fatty acids attached to the glycerol. One may be a saturated fatty acid and another a polyun-

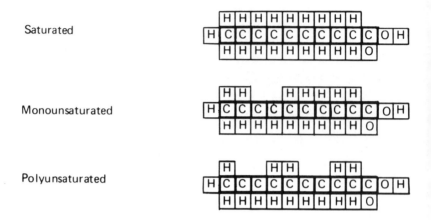

Fig. 21. The difference in saturated, monounsaturated, and polyunsaturated fat is in the number of missing hydrogen (H) blocks from the carbon (C) chain.

saturated fatty acid, or there may be two different saturated fatty acids and a monounsaturated fatty acid. The fat in your food is almost all triglycerides.

The fat in any one food is commonly a mixture of different amounts of the different fatty acids. In general the fat from mammal sources such as beef, pork, and lamb is about half saturated fat and half unsaturated fat. Although pork contains a little more polyunsaturated fat, the unsaturated fat in beef and lamb is mostly monounsaturated fatty acid. Be on your toes for food advertisements claiming a food is healthy because it contains a lot of unsaturated fat. Unless the unsaturated fat is polyunsaturated and not monounsaturated, there is no evidence that it is beneficial to your health. You can't expect to get much polyunsaturated fatty acid from beef, pork, or lamb.

Fatty acids vary according to the length of their carbon skeleton. Short-chain fatty acids have only four to six carbon blocks, medium-chain fatty acids have eight to ten, and long-chain fatty acids have twelve or more carbon blocks. The number of carbon blocks is usually an even number, four, six, eight, or more in man.

Would you like to know what your fat contains? The human fat tissue contains at least twenty-four long-chain fatty acids. Only seven of these, however, constitute over 91 per cent of the fatty acids.

Major Fatty Acids in Human Fat

Oleic (monounsaturated—18 carbons)	43.1%
Palmitic (saturated—16 carbons)	19.0
Linoleic (polyunsaturated—18 carbons)	13.9
Stearic (saturated—18 carbons)	6.2
Palmitic (monounsaturated—16 carbons)	5.1
Myristic (saturated—14 carbons)	3.5
Lauric (saturated—12 carbons)	0.9

By category, 29.6 per cent of your fatty acids are saturated, 48.2 per cent monounsaturated, and 13.9 per cent polyunsaturated.

In most of the foods we eat the majority of unsaturated fatty acids are oleic acid and linoleic acid. Fish oils, however, commonly have long chains with more than two spots on the carbon chain where pairs of hydrogen blocks are missing. The principal one of these is linoleic acid, containing eighteen carbon blocks with three locations where pairs of hydrogen blocks are missing.

I get a lot of questions about terms used in describing fats on food labels. Partially hydrogenated means additional hydrogen blocks have been added to unsaturated fatty acids. This process converts an unsaturated fat into a saturated fat. Saturated fats produced by this process are no better than saturated fats normally occurring in meat and a variety of animal products. The term "hardened" also refers to hydrogenating unsaturated fatty acids. Many unsaturated fats are liquid at room temperature. Saturated fats, like tallow, are often solid. Converting an unsaturated fat to a saturated fat causes it to be more solid or "hardened."

Among the thousands of misleading or incorrect statements made about fats is the claim that heating polyunsaturated fats converts them into saturated fats. Heating the oils may split the fatty acid from the glycerol unit but that has nothing to do with converting the oil to a saturated fat. Cooking oils have been used for centuries by the populations of the world with the lowest incidence of heart and vascular disease.

The fat in our food is one of the biggest sources of our calories. Not only does a gram of fat contain over twice as many calories as a gram of protein or carbohydrate, but there is usually very little water or bulk in our food fat. The fatty tissue in animals is less than 20 per cent water. Contrast this to lean muscle tissue which is over 70 per cent water. The difference in calorie value for fat and protein plus the water factor means that *there are about as many calories in a pound of fat as there are in five pounds of lean meat.* This point is also important in terms of weight control and obesity problems that I'll discuss after explaining the basic metabolic concepts.

Most people are unaware how widespread fat calories are in their food. It is beyond the scope of this presentation to give you a listing of the fat content of most common foods. I have included detailed tables of values for this purpose in an earlier book, *What You Need to Know about Food and Cooking for Health,* and you can consult those tables for more details.

About 80 per cent of the weight of butter is fat, the rest is water. Butter and the butterfat in all dairy products are over 56 per cent saturated fat, about 33 per cent monosaturated fat, and less than 3 per cent poly-unsaturated fat. For this reason many heart specialists have recommended using one of the soft margarines. You can get soft tub margarines containing only 17 per cent saturated fat and over 38 per cent polyunsaturated fat. A trick I've learned is to mix thoroughly two tubs of soft margarine with one tub of a polyunsaturated oil. I use safflower oil. Add a half teaspoon of imitation-butter-flavored salt. The mixture will be almost liquid. If you want it to be creamy like butter you can store it in the freezing compartment of your refrigerator.

Of the common cooking oils, safflower oil has the least saturated fat (8 per cent) and the most polyunsaturated fat (72 per cent). Corn oil is next (10 per cent saturated fat and 53 per cent polyunsaturated fat). Olive oil is low in saturated fat (11 per cent) but also low in polyunsaturated fat (7 per cent). You should be particularly cautious about coconut oil, often called vegetable oil on food labels. It is 86 per cent saturated fat. If you want to avoid saturated fats you need to avoid coconut oil and all food products containing it. What if the label is not specific and just states vegetable oil? Assume it is coconut oil and get a product that is better labeled.

As you can guess from what I said about coconut oil and olive oil, not all foods of plant origin are low in fat or even saturated fat. About 88 per cent of the calories in baking chocolate are fat and over half of this is saturated fat.

The cereals contain a small amount of fat. As an example, 5 per cent of the calories in whole-wheat flour and nearly 4 per cent of the calories in wheat flakes are fat. Of course, if you use a product like wheat germ a fourth of the calories are fat, but only a fifth of these are saturated fat while nearly half are polyunsaturated.

Of the cheese group, only one-third of the calories in creamed cottage cheese are from fat. Only about 3 per cent of the calories are fat in uncreamed cottage cheese. But most cheeses, cheddar being a good example, are over 70 per cent fat calories and over half of that is saturated fat.

About half of the fat in whole milk and cream is saturated fat. Many of the substitutes, particularly the powdered cream substitute products, are made with coconut oil and almost all of their high fat content is saturated fat.

Commercial white bread contains 11 per cent fat calories. The fat calories in biscuits vary from 15 to 50 per cent of the total calories. The flakier varieties have the highest fat content. You can make low-fat biscuits from special recipes. Saltine crackers are 25 per cent fat calories. Commercial dinner rolls vary from 25 to 50 per cent fat and sweet rolls are commonly 50 per cent fat calories.

Many of the sauces and salad dressings contain an appreciable amount of polyunsaturated fat, but their total fat content is high. A few of these are barbecue sauce, 67 per cent fat calories; mayonnaise, 97 per cent fat calories; mustard, 46 per cent fat calories; salad dressings, 92 per cent fat calories.

Many people are surprised to learn that vegetables contain calories from fat. Cooked broccoli contains 10 per cent fat calories; greens, 13 per cent; cooked sweet corn, 10 per cent; Boston lettuce, 11 per cent; red chili peppers, 21 per cent; dill pickles, 15 per cent; and tomatoes, 8 per cent. This isn't a lot but it shows how widespread fat calories are in your foods.

Even fruit contains fat. Examples are apples, 9 per cent; blackberries, 12 per cent; cranberries, 13 per cent; grapes (American), 12 per cent; raspberries, 16 per cent; strawberries, 11 per cent.

Fish is a good source of polyunsaturated fat. As a rule of thumb, you can consider the fat in fish about one-third saturated, one-third monounsaturated, and one-third polyunsaturated. The amount of fat in fish varies tremendously. The percentage of the calories from fat may be quite high even though the amount of fat is small, because many fish are low-calorie foods with over 80 per cent of their weight as water. Some values of fat in the fish group are: cod, 3.5 per cent; catfish (fresh-water), 27.2 per cent; flounder and sole, 9 per cent; drum, 40 per cent; pompano, 52 per cent; canned salmon, 50 per cent; and lake trout, 55 per cent.

The amount of fat in poultry also varies widely. As a rule, the younger bird contains the least fat. A fryer contains much less fat than a roaster, a young turkey, less than a mature bird. The light meat is much lower in fat, and much of the fat is in the skin. In general, about a third of the fat is saturated fat and a fifth is polyunsaturated.

I have already mentioned beef. Its fat is about half saturated fat and a little less than half monounsaturated. It contains very little polyunsaturated fat. Again the percentage of the calories from fat varies tremendously. About the lowest fat content is in the separable lean of round steak, about 5 per cent by weight, but that's 31 per cent of its calories as fat. By contrast, over 80 per cent of the calories in a choice Porterhouse steak are from fat.

Pork usually contains a lot of fat, though there are some lean cuts of ham. Generally, one-third of the fat is saturated, a little less than half is monounsaturated, and 10 per cent is polyunsaturated.

The cold cuts, such as bologna and frankfurters, and sausage are 80 per cent fat and much of that is saturated.

Baked desserts are usually high in fat. Over 40 per cent of the calories in a commercial devil's-food cake are fat. Cookies, pies, and puddings contain a great deal of fat. There are a few exceptions, such as angel-food cake. You can prepare your own baked goods from special recipes, however, and greatly reduce the amount of fat. By using a polyunsaturated oil you can drastically cut down the amount of saturated fat in such foods.

How much fat should you eat a day? As with carbohydrates, that depends a lot on what else you eat. Your body needs a minimal number of calories (energy) a day, and the two big sources of calories are carbohydrates and fat. The one major purpose of fat in the diet is to provide calories, and that means energy for the body functions. You will need some fat just to absorb the fat-soluble vitamins from the intestinal tract, but you don't need much for that. There is enough fat in the foods you normally eat, even if you eat only cereals, vegetables, and fruit (which I don't recommend) to absorb vitamins. Of course, if you have pancreatic disease or one of the diseases affecting absorption from the intestine, you might have a problem.

As you can see from the comments on the fat content of a variety of foods, the real problem is how to avoid fats. You can hardly avoid having some fat in the diet. As a guide you should probably plan to limit your calories from fat to about one-third of your total calories and limit the calories from saturated fat to about 10 per cent of your total calories. For a guide to the calories from fat and methods of low-fat cooking you can use my book *What You Need to Know about Food and Cooking for Health*.

There is some evidence that you need small amounts of the polyunsaturated fats in your diet for normal growth and body function. The principal one is linoleic acid, a common fatty acid in cereals, cooking oils, vegetables, fish, and poultry. Some of the fatty acids can be converted to other fatty acids in the body. This is not a free-for-all exchange, however. One fatty acid can be converted only to a limited number of other fatty acids so they are interchangeable only within groups.

The animal species characteristics do control to a considerable extent what kind of fatty acids will make up the fat deposits, and man is no exception. You can, however, affect the composition of fat deposits to some extent by the kind of fatty acids in the diet. The amount of polyunsaturated fat in pork can be increased and recently there has been some evidence that cattle fed special foods tend to have more polyunsaturated fat in their fat depots. Again, we see the truth of the statement that you are what you eat.

The fat in your various foods exerts its first important role in the stomach. Fats tend to delay the emptying of the stomach. If you want to slow down the absorption of anything you should take it after ingesting fat. This is why it takes longer for alcohol to have an effect on a person after he has consumed some fat than it would otherwise. Some fat may still be in the stomach as long as twenty-four hours after it was ingested. Individuals who have reactive low blood glucose caused by rapid emptying of the stomach often do better if their diet contains more fat. This helps spread out the time for stomach emptying and levels off the amount of glucose in the blood, avoiding the peak and valley effects that cause all the trouble.

Fat is absorbed in the small intestine, but only with the aid of bile salts and the enzyme lipase from the pancreas. The bile salts emulsify or increase the solubility of the fat particles and the lipase splits the fat into glycerol and fatty acids. There is some dispute over how far the splitting goes but in any case the fat that finally enters the intestinal cells is not in the same form as when you ingested it. Once the fat is inside the cell it is again acted upon. The end result is to connect several triglyceride units of fat with a protein. Fats are not soluble in water so they can't dissolve in blood. Proteins are water soluble so nature solves the problem by hooking the fat to a protein, making a soluble fat particle.

Each fat particle formed contains a variety of fats. There will be unsaturated fatty acids, saturated fatty acids, and those mysterious fats called phospholipids. The term lipid means fat or fatlike. Not all lipids are really fats. A fatty acid attached to a chemical unit containing phosphorus is called a phospholipid. They are more soluble than ordinary fatty acids because of the solubility of the phosphorus unit. The fat–protein particle also contains variable amounts of cholesterol. Cholesterol is a typical lipid which is not a fat. Technically an alcohol, it is made up of twenty-seven blocks of carbon, and because of its size it is a solid waxy material. The whole particle of triglycerides, cholesterol, and protein is called a chylomicron. As these accumulate in the wall of the small intestine, they cause the intestine to turn a waxy white color which remains until all of the fat has moved through the intestinal wall.

A few small or short-chain fatty acids that are freed in this process pass directly into the veins and are carried immediately to the liver. The vast majority of the fat in your food, though, ends up as chylomicrons and passes through the intestinal wall into the lymphatic circulation. They give the normally clear lymph a milky characteristic. Through the lymph the fatty particles are channeled into the bloodstream just before the blue unoxygenated blood returns to the heart. Once in the blood they may give it a milky appearance. Substances in the blood act as clearing agents to break down these large particles and get them stored.

The smaller fat particles are literally absorbed into the fat cells and the liver. The fat cells are those special cells used to store all the fat we accumulate, process it, and release it when we need it. We all have them, but the fat cells in an obese person contain a lot more fat than those in a thinner person. As you lose weight you don't lose fat cells, they only decrease in size.

A small amount of free fatty acids in the blood are hooked on to albumin, an important protein in the blood. This makes them soluble. They can be picked up by other cells in the body and used for energy.

The liver is the great fat processor. As the fat is released from fat cells, it is circulated to the liver for processing. It can convert the fat it receives into different forms. It is the principal place where fat is broken down to ketones (more about that later). The liver makes fat from other foods, and it makes most of the cholesterol generated in your body. It has a lot to do with regulating the amount of new fat particles, combinations of triglycerides, phospholipids, cholesterol, and protein, in the blood. These are smaller than the chylomicron and will not make the blood milky. They are called lipoproteins.

The size of the lipoprotein is thought to be important in causing fatty deposits in the arteries. The larger ones (not chylomicrons, however) are the important ones. Apparently the larger the particle the more triglyceride units there are for each protein unit. The larger particles tend to contain more saturated fat, less phospholipid, more cholesterol, and as a result are less soluble than smaller lipoproteins.

The lipoproteins are classified on the basis of their size. The small ones are called alpha lipoproteins, the larger ones beta lipoproteins. It follows that if a person has a lot of beta lipoproteins in his blood he is more likely to have atherosclerosis with its complications of heart attacks, strokes, and other medical problems. The various examinations that doctors perform are directed toward evaluating this tendency. The cholesterol measurement provides some information on how many of these larger particles you have. The higher the cholesterol the greater the number of beta lipoproteins. The cholesterol measurement has proved to be quite satisfactory for this purpose in clinical use. The measurement of the triglycerides is also an attempt to assess the number and character of the fatty particles in the blood. Other more sophisticated tests are also used, but they all come back to the central point of evaluating the amount and type of fatty-cholesterol-containing particles in the blood.

The liver seems to have definite limitations on the amount of fat it can process. You'll see evidence of this in starvation, diabetes, and problems that require the liver to process enormous amounts of fat. The fat accumulates in excess amounts in the liver and damages it. The liver also produces fewer of the large fatty particles that cause atherosclerosis if the diet is low in fat and low in saturated fat. For complicated reasons the liver seems to produce less cholesterol and big fatty particles if a reasonable part of the limited fat intake is polyunsaturated fat.

Many factors influence how the liver processes fat, including the sex hormones. That is why the liver in childbearing women commonly produces less cholesterol and small, less important fat particles. Men, on the other hand, tend to produce excess amounts of cholesterol-containing large fatty particles. As a result men have heart attacks and strokes much earlier than women.

8

FAT TO ENERGY, ENERGY TO FAT

The fats you can use for energy or cell activity are in the form of triglyceride units. They are carried by the bloodstream to the various body cells for use as energy. It really doesn't matter whether the triglycerides come from what you have just eaten or have been released from the fat cells. They all go through the same process.

Within the cell the first step is to tear the glycerol loose from the three fatty acids. This process requires the hydrogen and oxygen building blocks of water. Glycerol, you remember, is a three-carbon chain containing three units of water and two additional blocks of hydrogen. It is very much like a carbohydrate. In fact, by adding to it a unit of phosphate energy from ATP, the glycerol is converted to PGA, the combination of a phosphate unit and glycerol. I mentioned this in the discussion of the breakdown of glucose. At this stage the glycerol is equivalent to a half unit of glucose and follows the same process as glucose. Yes, it can either be converted to blood glucose or go to pyruvic acid and finally be used for energy like any other three-carbon unit from glucose. From 100 grams of triglyceride fat the body can make 12 grams of blood glucose from its glycerol units. In the final analysis, fat can contribute to the blood-glucose level, to a limited extent, from glycerol.

The fatty acids are the big source of fat energy. Most of them contain sixteen or eighteen carbon blocks. A great deal of energy is used to bind these blocks together. The breakdown of the fatty-acid chain is accomplished by using Co-A, the high-energy coenzyme. The Co-A literally hooks on to the end of the fatty acid.

Through the use of the coenzyme NAD as a hydrogen carrier along the familiar hydrogen express, excess hydrogen unites with oxygen to form water. The end two-carbon blocks attached to Co-A break off, and a new unit of Co-A hooks on to the end of the carbon chain. In this way the carbon chain is literally chopped off in two-carbon segments, one after another, just as if you were slicing salami.

The two-carbon unit attached to Co-A should not be a stranger to you. It is active acetate, a major product in the final part of the processing of glucose. This is the point when the processing of fatty acids joins the common processing line for glucose. The active acetate gives up acetic acid which joins with four-carbon OAA to form citric acid. It is then processed along the same energy circle, giving up two units of carbon dioxide, equivalent to the two-carbon blocks in acetic acid. In the process it is stripped of its energy.

How much energy is involved? A six-carbon segment from the fatty acid, comparable to the glucose's six-carbon segment, yields three units of acetic acid. In processing them to carbon dioxide they yield enough energy to form forty-four ATP units. Remember, a unit of glucose yields only thirty-eight units of ATP.

You need some OAA to form the citric acid to complete the energy cycle. This comes from pyruvic acid. As long as you have enough OAA you can process the active acetate without any difficulty. Of course, you can use the glycerol to form the pyruvic acid and finally the OAA. Nevertheless, in the absence of glucose, processing fat is not as readily accomplished.

Under certain conditions, most of them abnormal, as in fasting, the fats may form ketone bodies. You may have heard a lot about them from past popularized diet regimes. An excess amount of ketone bodies can upset the body chemistry and cause serious problems. They also tend to accumulate in untreated severe diabetes. In large amounts they can cause coma and even death. Almost all of the ketone bodies are formed in the liver. The basic ketone body is acetoacetic acid, simply a combination of two units of acetic acid. It can lose two hydrogen blocks and exist in a slightly different form (beta hydroxy butyric acid), or it can lose a unit of carbon dioxide to become three-carbon acetone. The acetone formation occurs primarily in the lungs as the excess unit of carbon dioxide is lost. The acetone exhaled by the lungs imparts an alcoholic smell to the breath. The alcohol smell has caused many a diabetic on the verge of coma to be jailed, suspected of being drunk. This is a real tragedy since the diabetic in this state is in need of emergency medical treatment, not a trip to the jail.

The ketone bodies that are not lost through the lungs or processed for

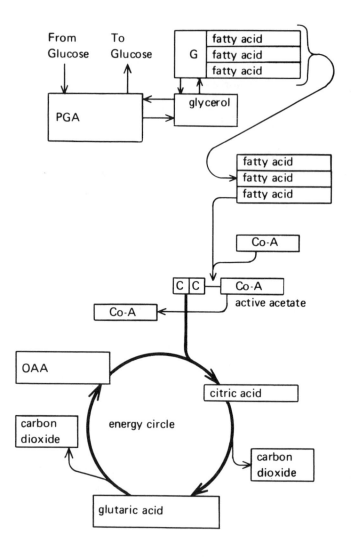

Fig. 22. The breakdown of fats.

energy are lost in the urine. Don't believe those wild claims that by inducing ketosis you can lose a lot of weight. Unless you are sick, you won't lose enough ketone bodies to help that much.

Although neither the liver nor some brain cells can use the ketone bodies, other tissue cells can, up to a point. The first step is to convert the

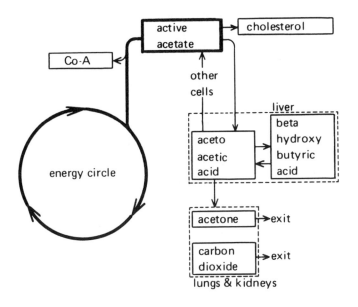

Fig. 23. The relationship of active acetate to the formation of ketone bodies and cholesterol.

acetoacetic acid back to two-carbon active acetate. It can then be processed through the ordinary energy cycle with OAA to be broken down to carbon dioxide and yield energy. This requires oxygen, and, unless there is sufficient oxygen and OAA, the process cannot be accomplished. When enormous amounts of ketones are formed or when they can't be utilized, they build up in the bloodstream and coma may follow. This is what happens in diabetic coma.

Since dismantling fat yields energy it shouldn't surprise you that the formation of fat sops up energy. Your body fat is literally energy in the bank. This includes the energy stripped from carbohydrates, proteins, and alcohol we don't need. It follows that fat can be, and is, formed from carbohydrates, protein, and alcohol, as well as the fat in our food.

The process begins with active acetate. This location on the processing line is a main intersection of the metabolic activities. Not much happens in the energy exchange system that doesn't involve active acetate, the two-carbon bit attached to Co-A. Don't think of fat formation as simply a reversal of dismantling fat. It is not. Although the multiple steps and enzymes involved are complex, the total reaction can be summarized quite simply. To a number of two-carbon active acetate units add some carbon dioxide units and some hydrogen, carried by the coenzyme NADP (NADP.H), and provide some energy from ATP. Presto, the active ace-

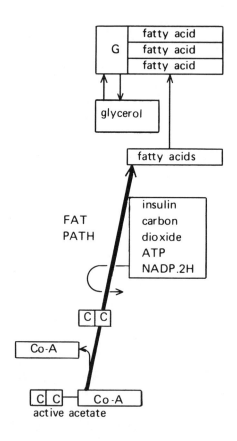

Fig. 24. The use of active acetate in the formation of fat.

tate units are joined end to end in a long chain. The hydrogen blocks are transferred from the NADP.H to the carbon skeleton to fill up the carbon chain with hydrogen blocks.

The energy that is trapped with the hydrogen blocks attached to NADP.H is transferred to the newly formed fatty acid. The ATP breaks down to provide energy to bind the active-acetate units end to end. Energy is also sopped up when active acetate breaks down to simple acetic acid. The Co-A previously attached to the acetic acid to form active acetate is then free to be involved in another transaction. It takes just as much energy to build fat as it does to tear it down. Each unit of fat then literally absorbs energy from ATP in its formation.

Keep in mind that since fat is formed from the building units of active acetate and since active acetate is formed by the processing of carbohydrate, protein, alcohol, and fat, body fat can be formed from any of these foods. It is completely untrue that protein makes you slim. It isn't *which calories* you eat that counts in terms of forming fat deposits, it is *how many calories* you eat. Once it is formed, fat is fat regardless of whether it comes from fat, carbohydrate, protein, or alcohol.

There is another interesting observation. The formation of fat uses the coenzyme NADP, but tearing down fatty acids uses NAD. Tearing down fat liberates hydrogen blocks that must be transported by NAD to unite with oxygen to form water. Building fat uses hydrogen blocks transported by NADP. A very interesting trick can happen here. The hydrogen blocks transported by NAD in tearing down carbohydrates, fat, and protein can be picked up by NADP and used to form fatty acids. This means oxygen is not needed to unload the hydrogen from NAD if you are using hydrogen to form fat. In short, by forming fat a cell can process food we eat without requiring a lot of oxygen we normally need to release energy. This may be a very important factor in explaining why some overweight people always feel tired. Their cells use the "no oxygen" processing route (fat path) to form fat rather than the "high oxygen" route to release energy (energy circle). Why does this occur? The reasons are not entirely clear, but perhaps the amount of oxygen actually delivered to the cell is an important factor. And this may get back to adequate circulation. If your circulation isn't delivering enough oxygen to the cells the best the cell can do may be to form fat to process food rather than release energy.

Certainly exercise increases circulation and oxygen delivery. At the same time it requires energy. One possible benefit from exercise may be to stimulate our cells to use the energy-releasing energy circle rather than the energy-storing fat path. This may also offer an explanation why an inactive person feels tired—he is forming fat, not energy, because his circulation is not stimulated by exercise. Then, with a little exercise after a sedentary day in the office, there is a sudden surge in energy. Resting simply makes matters worse.

There are many possible ways the body can influence whether food is used for energy or takes the fat path. Women tend to have more fat stores than active men. Female hormones apparently stimulate cells to process food along the fat path to maintain characteristic female fat pads. Male hormones evidently do the opposite, and that is why men tend to have muscular, lean bodies. Castration of male animals stimulates using the fat path rather than the energy circle. Among the secrets of stimulating the body to use the energy circle as opposed to the fat path is probably the ideal way to have lots of energy and not get fat. Considering the amount of rich food we are all capable of eating, we should all be turned into human energy dynamos, if we only knew the secrets. I suspect that this is the real reason why some thin people are so energetic. Their system, for unexplained reasons, tends to use the energy-yielding circle rather than the fat-forming path. These people tend to eat a lot, never get fat, and have lots of energy. We all know people like that.

The formation of fat can occur in the fat cells, liver, and many other body cells. It is facilitated by insulin. Experiments have shown that liver slices treated with insulin will speed up the process of fatty acid formation markedly. The opposite also occurs. The diabetic rat liver slices, without insulin action, cannot form fatty acids. These reactions also fit with the clinical observation that patients who have a true overproduction of insulin tend to have more fat deposits and obesity problems, whereas a severe diabetic, not adequately treated, tends to have trouble forming fat. I'll discuss other important factors in the diabetic later.

Fatty acids do not remain unattached in the body. They are joined to glycerol to form mono-, di-, and triglycerides, mostly the latter. Phosphoglyceraldehyde (PGA), the three-carbon unit with phosphorus formed from glucose, gives up its phosphate unit and is converted to glycerol. The glycerol can then unite with the fatty acids. Since this part of the carbohydrate processing system is reversible it follows that PGA used to make glycerol can come from either pyruvic acid or glucose.

A large part of the cholesterol in our bodies is manufactured by the liver. It, too, is built from that magic unit, active acetate. In a series of complex steps the active acetate is disconnected from Co-A and the energy used to unite all twenty-seven carbon building blocks into cholesterol. Because of the number of carbon blocks used and the way they are arranged, cholesterol is a large unit. Since active acetate comes from fat, carbohydrate, protein, and even alcohol, it follows that the carbon blocks from any of these foods can end up in the formation of cholesterol.

What you eat does make a difference, though, in relation to cholesterol formation. The amount of cholesterol produced depends primarily on the liver cell actions. For some unexplained reason the liver tends to form more cholesterol if the diet contains a lot of fat, particularly saturated fat. Just eating more calories than you need for energy from any and all types of food favors the formation of larger amounts of cholesterol. That's why it's important to watch your total calorie intake if you want to keep your cholesterol down. Just don't get fat.

The liver has a lot to do with forming fatty acids for triglycerides, controlling whether the fatty acids are made up of saturated or unsaturated fatty acids, and how these are joined with proteins to form lipoproteins. It follows that the liver is the great regulator of how many and what type of lipoproteins are in your blood. It is equally true that the liver regulates, to a large extent, how much cholesterol is in your blood. But never be misled by this statement. What the liver does to accomplish this depends primarily on your living habits, diet, and exercise, as well as other factors. You can influence the function of the liver in producing cholesterol and lipoproteins by what you eat.

A significant amount of cholesterol is also formed in the cells lining the intestine. The cholesterol in the blood really represents the cholesterol you consume in your food, that produced in the intestinal wall, and that formed in the liver. The cholesterol formed in the liver amounts to one or two thousand milligrams a day (one or two grams). This is far in excess of what most people get in their diet, but the dietary intake varies tremendously. An egg yolk may contain from 255 to 275 milligrams. There is cholesterol, usually in lesser amounts, in many other animal foods. It is easy to consume 600 or 700 milligrams of cholesterol a day. The Inter-Society Commission on Heart Disease recommends that we limit our daily cholesterol intake to 300 milligrams.

The cholesterol formed in the liver is dumped into the bile and flows

Cholesterol Content of Some Common Foods (in milligrams)

Beef, lamb, pork (3½ oz.—100 grams)	70
Chicken (3½ oz.—100 grams)	60
Fish (3½ oz.—100 grams)	25–70
Liver (3½ oz.—100 grams)	300
Butter (1 tablespoon)	30
Margarine (vegetable)	0
Milk, whole (1 cup)	27
skim (1 cup)	8
Cheese, cheddar (3½ oz.—100 grams)	100
cream (3½ oz.—100 grams)	120
cottage (3½ oz.—100 grams)	15
Egg yolk (one)	250
whole egg (one)	250
egg white	0
Vegetables, fruits, cereals	0

with it through the bile duct into the small intestine. Here it mixes with the cholesterol in the diet and is no longer distinguishable from diet cholesterol. Cholesterol is cholesterol no matter where it comes from. Most of the mixed pool of cholesterol in the small intestine is absorbed into the intestinal wall. More cholesterol can be formed here, and the final amount is then passed with fat into the lymph channels and finally into the blood. About 300 to 1000 milligrams of cholesterol are eliminated with the rest of the food residue from the bowel each day. If more cholesterol is being absorbed back into the bloodstream than the body is eliminating, you will begin to have a rise in cholesterol in your blood. This can be the result of overproduction of cholesterol or eating too much cholesterol or a combination of both.

The bile salts needed to emulsify fat for its absorption come from cholesterol. The liver converts some cholesterol to bile salts. These pass with the cholesterol-containing bile into the small intestine and perform their role in the absorption of fat. They are reabsorbed, go back via the circulation to the liver, and are used again and again. Ordinarily they are recirculated five to ten times before they are destroyed.

Cholesterol is also the basic substance used to form some of our vital hormones, called the steroid hormones. These include the adrenal hormones and the sex hormones. It takes but a very small amount of cholesterol to form sufficient amounts of these substances. You needn't worry that a low cholesterol count will impair the formation of these important hormones.

What is the normal amount of cholesterol in the blood? Opinions vary, but a frequently quoted range is 150 to 250 (milligrams in a tenth of a liter of blood serum). Studies on heart attacks and atherosclerosis suggest that to be in the best risk group, as far as these problems are concerned, a value of less than 220 is desirable.

9

WHAT ARE PROTEINS?

There is probably more confusion about proteins than any other food. Some people eat lots of protein thinking this will help them lose weight or stay slim. Others guzzle down protein powders and protein pills of all descriptions in hopes of gaining weight. Obviously something is amiss here.

Let's start out with the understanding that proteins are simply amino acids connected together. You can think of amino acids as the building blocks of proteins. Incidentally, we know what the amino acids are that make up all the proteins of the body and the body hormones, enzymes, and other secretions. They have been defined down to their last building block and how the blocks are arranged. When several amino acids are connected it is called a polypeptide; a protein is made up of several polypeptides.

You may be surprised to know that the body uses only about twenty different amino acids to build body protein, and in all there are only about twenty-five amino acids. Some of these are made from other amino acids, and this accounts for the different number of amino acids listed by different authorities. There are fewer amino acids used to build our proteins than there are letters in the alphabet to build our words. Think of amino acids as letters and proteins as words.

A protein may contain literally hundreds of amino-acid units connected in a variety of ways and different sequences. This is what makes a protein complicated. Some proteins are made up of relatively few amino acids. Most of the body proteins contain fifteen or eighteen different amino acids. Insulin, the hormone that prevents diabetes, is built out of fifty-one amino-acid units. So it is not difficult to define what our protein is made from, only a problem of knowing how all of the building blocks are put together.

Did you know that even your memory and knowledge appear to depend on amino acids? It has already been reported that a rat's memory of the sound of an electric bell is a simple combination of six amino acids. You can inject the six-amino-acid unit into other rats not trained to recognize the bell, and then they will also recognize the sound of the bell. The implications are obvious. The intellectual processes appear to be dependent on the use of amino acids to form specific chains of proteins within the brain.

Part of the confusion about proteins arises from the fact that amino acids can be used either for energy, just as fats and carbohydrates are, or as the building blocks to build muscle, blood, and a variety of important body proteins. You can use a simple analogy here to building a house. You can use boards for the walls of the house and in this way they become part of the structure, but you can also use the boards for fuel in the fireplace to provide energy in the form of heat. It is the same with amino acids. They are building materials that can also be used to provide energy. For the most part, carbohydrates and fats are like oil and gas: they can heat the house but they can't be used to build it.

The similarity doesn't end there. If there is no fuel in the house you could chop down a wooden wall and burn the wood for heat energy. The body does just that. If there is no other source of energy available it will simply take the protein out of the muscles and use it for energy. We literally chop down our walls and use them for body fuel. This is an important concept because it means that the carbohydrate and fat in your diet spare the body the necessity of using amino acids for fuel and permits them to be saved for building processes. It is important to understand that the only way protein provides energy for the body is in the same way carbohydrates and fat do. They are disconnected into the basic blocks, allowing the energy bound in the amino acids to be stripped out and the building blocks discarded.

The amino acids are only a little different from the fatty acids. You need only to add the blocks used for ammonia to the carbon chain. The word amino really means ammonia. The amino unit consists of one block of nitrogen and two blocks of hydrogen (ammonia contains one nitrogen block and three hydrogen blocks). Amino acids are different from carbohydrates and fatty acids in that they contain nitrogen as well as carbon, hydrogen, and oxygen. It's that simple.

The simplest amino acid is glycine. It contains only two carbon blocks, five blocks of hydrogen, one block of nitrogen, and two blocks of oxygen. You can think of its block diagram as looking like Figure 25.

The next-simplest amino acid, alanine, just adds one more carbon block attached to three hydrogen blocks. You can picture it as in Figure 26.

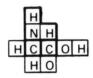

Fig. 25. A simplified block diagram
of the amino acid glycine.

Now you are set to form a lot of different amino acids simply by extending the length of the carbon chain. Not all the block arrangements are that simple. Some can be rather complex, but the underlying concept is the same. You are now down to the basic truth about the human body: it is composed mostly of water (hydrogen and oxygen), carbon, and a little nitrogen.

It's easy to see that carbohydrates come from the plant world's action on carbon dioxide and water. And it is easy to see that the carbohydrate can be converted to fat. But where does the nitrogen come from to fit into this life cycle requiring protein formation? It comes from the air. About

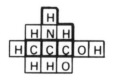

Fig. 26. A simplified block diagram
of the amino acid alanine.

80 per cent of the air around us is nitrogen. How does it get incorporated into animal tissue? The nitrogen is trapped in the soil and used by the plant in its growth.

There are two ways nitrogen gets into the soil, unless we deliberately add nitrogen, for example, in fertilizer. The soil will trap nitrogen from the air as a result of the action of sunlight on the air and soil. This works better if the surface of the soil is rough and exposed. Farmers have known for centuries that they grow better crops if a field is plowed and the broken earth left unplanted for a season. This is not as effective, though, as using legumes such as alfalfa, clover, soybeans, or any of the bean family. These plants literally pull nitrogen out of the air and deposit it in the roots within the soil. This is the basis for crop rotation. A poor cornfield can be converted to alfalfa for a number of years, then it can be used again to produce a good yield of corn. From nitrogen in the soil to protein for us, there are two main routes. We can eat the vegetable products that contain proteins, such as beans, or the animals that process the vegetable products containing protein to form animal protein.

The body is pretty sneaky in handling our amino acids. It can rip off the amino blocks of nitrogen and hydrogen and give them to another carbon chain to form a new amino acid. This robbing-Peter-to-pay-Paul tactic is called transamination. The big ripoff occurs in the liver. In addition, the body can change one amino acid into another, and, within limits, it can take nitrogen from another source and manufacture a new amino acid. It isn't surprising, then, that your body can take carbohydrate and fat and use parts of them in building new amino acids and eventually protein. You should not be misled, however. To accomplish this sleight-of-hand exercise the body needs a ready supply of amino acids. You cannot meet your protein requirement by eating just carbohydrates or fat.

There are some amino acids the body cannot manufacture from other amino acids or other nutrients. These must be supplied in your food if you are to maintain life and health. These are called the essential amino acids. Other names have been suggested for them, but the old term "essential" has stuck, and you will see it on a lot of food labels. If the diet is totally lacking in these you will die. They are essential for growth, maintenance, and reproduction. Yes, there is some truth in the idea that you need protein for a satisfactory sex life. Just don't expect that taking more than your body requires will do anything for you in that department.

Even adults need eight essential amino acids for maintenance of their body. Two more are needed for growth or any situation requiring the body to produce more protein, as in pregnancy. Muscle building is another case where more protein is needed, and that means more essential amino acids. In all then, for growth and maintenance, there are ten amino acids you need in your diet. These ten all have difficult names, but you need to have a list of them you can use for reference to food labels. They are every bit as important as the list of vitamins you probably already know. And, like vitamins, they cannot be manufactured in the body.

The Ten Essential Amino Acids

Valine	Phenylalanine
Leucine	Tryptophan
Isoleucine	Lysine
Threonine	Arginine
Methionine	Histidine

Of these, arginine and histidine are manufactured in sufficient amount in the body for ordinary maintenance, but the body cannot produce enough for growth requirements or situations which demand protein building processes.

It is important to understand that the body cannot build many of its structures or vital protein substances without these essential amino acids. It is similar to baking a cake. If you want to bake a chocolate cake and find you have no sugar, having all the flour and chocolate in the world won't help you. You can't do it. Similarly, you can eat an enormous amount of protein and unless it has enough essential amino-acid ingredients you can't build the needed proteins.

The rest of the amino acids in your food that are used for either energy or building are:

Nonessential Amino Acids

Alanine	Glutamine
Aspartic acid	(from glutamic acid)
Asparagine	Hydroxyproline
(from aspartic acid)	Proline
Cysteine	Serine
Cystine	Tyrosine
Glycine	Thyroxine and Triiodothyronine
Glutamic acid	(derivatives of tyrosine)

These are called the nonessential amino acids. This doesn't mean the body doesn't need them. They are "essential" in the sense that if you don't have enough of them for building materials there isn't going to be any building. All of these, though, can be manufactured from various other amino acids, and in a sense are at least partially interchangeable in providing the body's protein needs. It does take energy to form new amino acids from old, and it is better from a nutritional point of view to have an abundant amount of each of the amino acids in the body.

Your body can use the essential amino acids to manufacture the nonessential amino acids needed in the building process. If you do this, though, your requirement for essential amino acids goes way up. Using the analogy of building a house, you can use unfinished lumber for the framework and use the more expensive finished lumber for the interior of the walls. You can't, or at least you shouldn't if you want smooth walls, use the unfinished lumber for the interior surface. You could use finished lumber to build the framework, but that would be rather expensive. You should think of the essential amino acids as finished lumber: you can use them for anything, but you ought to save them for the places where you need them. The unfinished lumber you can use only in places you won't need to paint; this is comparable to the nonessential amino acids.

Even so, you need enough lumber for your building project. So it is with amino acids—you need enough total amino acids—total protein—to do the job. Just how much is enough? There is considerable variation, but it is generally agreed now that most adults need less than 70 grams of protein a day to maintain the body in good condition. This is a generous figure since many people get by and stay in good health on much less. These are the 1973 Recommended Daily Allowance (RDA) values:

Recommended Daily Allowance of Protein

Children	1–3 years	23 grams
	4–6 years	30
	7–10 years	36
Males	11–14 years	44
	15–18 years	54
	19–22 years	54
	over 22 years	56
Females	11–14 years	44
	15–18 years	48
	over 18 years	46
	pregnancy	add 30
	lactation	add 20

More is needed during growth conditions. Teenage boys during the years they are growing muscles will need more protein. Some may require as much as 100 grams of protein a day. If you use the generalization of 4 calories per gram of protein, that means 400 calories of their daily intake should be protein. During pregnancy and nursing a baby and when a person is growing muscles, for example in a body-building program, the protein requirements are increased.

Regarding muscles, you can get an idea of how much the body has to add to its protein content by using lean beef as a guide. There are 6 grams of protein in each ounce of separable lean muscle fibers of round steak. Expressed another way, about one-fifth of the weight of lean muscle fibers is from protein. It follows that for each pound of muscle fiber (not fat) gained a person will need to store about 100 grams of protein. A young man gaining a pound of muscle a week then will need to add 100 grams of protein (15 grams a day) to his body. Since not all protein is equally usable this probably means that he should increase his protein intake about 30 grams a day. It follows that his daily protein intake should be 70 to 100 grams a day to support his muscle growth requirements.

It is not enough to say how much protein a day a person needs. A minimal amount of the essential amino acids must be included. In general, a safe amount for an adult is from 1.5 to 2.5 grams of each of the essential amino acids a day. If you are in a building program, to be sure you have enough of everything you should provide the body with about twice that amount or 3 to 5 grams of each of the ten essential amino acids. It is unlikely that any program would result in a greater requirement than this.

What happens, then, if you do eat a lot more protein than you need? It is simple. The body just strips off the amino group and processes the carbon chain around the energy circle, just the same as fat or glucose, to release energy if you need it. Or the carbon skeleton can be processed along the fat path to store the energy as fat. Yes, excess protein simply becomes fat.

Now you can see the truth of the two extremes of the person who eats lots of protein to lose weight and the person who gobbles down protein powder in large amounts to gain weight. Eating protein while on a reducing diet ensures that you get all the amino acids you need and helps to protect against loss of body protein. But if the average person eats more protein than he needs for maintenance, the rest will be just calories no different from calories obtained from fats or carbohydrates. The individual trying to gain weight and eating more protein than his body needs for the building process will simply be using the excess protein as calories, no different from the calories in fats or carbohydrates.

The body can use only so much protein for building. The building process is stimulated by other factors unrelated to what you eat. A boy starts putting on muscle in adolescence because he is producing male hormone in large amounts. (The hormones that induce body growth are sometimes used by athletes for this purpose.) He uses more protein, then, to meet his expanded building requirements. The excess is used for energy or fat storage. If the hereditary characteristics call for growing lots of muscle then the protein will be used for that purpose. If they do not, the excess protein will not help. I like to compare this to building a house. If the building plans call for a brick wall, you can use only so many bricks. If you bring in an extra load of bricks it won't help at all, unless you change the fundamental building plan and increase the size of the wall.

In making sure you are getting enough protein in your diet for your metabolic needs you will encounter several terms on food labels. One of these is the note that the protein has been calculated by nitrogen content. The principle is fairly simple. It has been observed that 6.25 grams of protein contains 1 gram of nitrogen. By measuring the amount of nitrogen in the food, the amount of protein can be estimated. Actually, the amount of nitrogen in different proteins varies, but this is good enough for rough estimates. So when you see the notation ($N \times 6.25$) after protein on the label that's what it means.

Not all protein is easily digested and absorbed from the intestine. Proteins have been graded on their "coefficient of digestibility." The protein from animal sources, meat of mammals, fish, and poultry, is readily absorbed. It has a coefficient of 95 to 100 per cent. Wheat protein is almost as good. The protein in mature bean seeds is not nearly as good—only about 80 per cent.

Not all of the amino acids in the protein are used for building purposes. The utilization of the amino acids in a protein has also been studied. If the body tends to keep a lot of the amino acids, it is considered a quality protein. In general, the body is more apt to use all the protein in foods that have protein made of amino-acid grouping, much as in our body. For this reason the protein from the muscle of fish, poultry, and mammals is high-quality protein. It's more like the protein in our muscles than the bean protein is. Depending on its utilization and digestibility a protein is often graded as excellent, good, or poor. This is a somewhat misleading classification. A protein that is classified as poor may, nonetheless, be very useful in the diet. However, it usually requires more grams of protein to provide the growth and maintenance needs from foods containing poor protein than from foods containing excellent proteins.

The quality of a protein depends largely on the amino acids it contains. The value of various proteins has been studied by a clever method of using pure amino acids. Animals, and later heroic humans, were fed diets that contained everything the diet needed except protein. By adding or eliminating individual amino acids in the basic diet and studying growth, weight, and reproduction ability, the essential amino acids were identified and the amounts needed were determined. Proteins that contained sufficient amounts of all the amino acids to provide the protein needs when the rest of the diet was adequate were classified as complete proteins. These foods, in sufficient amounts, could meet all of an individual's protein requirements. Those proteins which did not contain all the needed amino acids were called incomplete proteins. You shouldn't get the idea that if a protein is incomplete it is not a good food. Quite the contrary; by using two different foods containing amino acids that complement each other, the amino-acid requirements can be met by incomplete proteins.

One of the classic experiments in nutrition involved the principle of using two incomplete proteins. Rats were fed only wheat, which is deficient in the essential amino acid lysine. Their growth rate was retarded on this diet. Another group was fed gelatin, which is deficient in a number of amino acids, but is rich in lysine. These rats also did poorly. When still another group of rats were fed the combination of the incomplete proteins they thrived. A diet of gelatin and wheat provided all the essential amino acids. Neither wheat nor gelatin alone would sustain the rats, but between them they did the job.

It should be noted here that some nutritionists bad-mouth gelatin as a "poor protein." So it is, in terms of utilization, and you would need to use a lot of it to provide a major portion of the body protein needs. This, however, doesn't detract from its usefulness in sufficient quantities to supplement a diet adequate in essential amino acids. The gelatin can be used to make up the total protein requirement. This is an important point because many patients can eat only small amounts of the foods that contain lots of complete proteins. A patient who cannot tolerate milk, or has a problem with cereals, or needs to restrict salt can get a lot of mileage by including gelatin in the diet.

Another recent experiment has received a lot of public attention. It was demonstrated that rats couldn't live on our white bread. So what is new? The wheat and gelatin experiment has been known for years. It is not expected that rats will live on bread alone—or man either. That is part of what a balanced diet is all about. Most of the breads are not known for their protein content anyway, and, as the classic experiment demonstrated, wheat protein is deficient in lysine, an essential amino acid. But that is not a scientific argument against the nutritive value of bread. Rather, white bread is a poor choice for nutrition because it is lacking in cereal fiber and roughage that is important to digestive functions.

Strict vegetarians who will not use any animal products, including eggs or milk, get all their needed amino acids from a combination of vegetables. Using beans, corn, and wheat in sufficient amount, you will get all the necessary amino acids. This is not a very good diet, however, for growing children or other conditions where growth is involved. It is better to include sufficient milk in the diet to improve the amount of protein in the food in these circumstances. The combination of beans and corn have kept many a civilization going in good health. The proteins complement each other. The different vitamins in them also help to provide the needed vitamin balance.

There is another curious fact about amino acids that you need to know. It has been claimed that to provide adequate protein intake you must have all the essential amino acids together in one meal. The idea is that building requires all the necessary parts and if one is missing you can't do the job—like trying to build a house without the materials for the roof. Although this idea is generally accepted, I have some doubts about how rigidly this needs to be applied to mature adults: In theory, our bodies should already contain the needed essential amino acids, and when our cells break down they are released into a common pool. These essential amino acids in our body are just as good as those in food—in fact, indistinguishable. I presume that these can be recycled. Even so, in a healthy diet there should be a number of foods that contain complete proteins. This would provide all the essential amino acids at one meal.

10

PROTEINS:
HOW MUCH? WHAT KIND?
WHERE TO GET THEM?

You may still be wondering how you are going to get all the protein you need in your diet, particularly since you must consider all those problems about essential and nonessential amino acids. It's not so difficult, but it will be helpful to look at the different food groups and see where they stand on protein content.

To get right down to the eating level, there are no proteins for you in sugars, syrups, jellies, jams, or honey. There aren't any in the fats or oils either. This includes butter, lard, margarine, and the cooking oils. These high-calorie foods haven't much to offer except calories. If you need calories because you do a lot of heavy labor, they are great. Otherwise— well, not so great. With the exception of the limited vitamin content of butter and margarine all of these foods deserve the label of "empty calories."

The cereal products are an important source of vitamins, and those that haven't been stripped of their roughage provide cereal fiber and bulk in the diet. They do contain some protein and it is fairly good protein. The problem is that you have to eat a lot of cereal to provide sufficient protein. Wheat protein is readily absorbed. As with other cereals, except corn and rice, it contains glutenin (gluten), a complete protein. It also contains a lot of incomplete protein and that is why rats fed only wheat failed to sustain growth. For individuals who must get all their protein from vegetable sources, gluten flour is a valuable product. Over 40 per cent of its weight is protein. Bread made from gluten flour, then, becomes a valuable source of protein.

A good way to express the protein content of food is to give the percentage of a food's weight that is protein. Obviously this is also grams of protein in each 100 grams of food. All you need to do, then, to find out how much protein there is in 4 ounces, a pound, or a kilogram of the food is to multiply its weight by the percentage of protein. If you want to know how many calories of protein that is, you can use the generalization of multiplying the grams of protein by four. That is not an exact figure but it is usable for most household diets. Meats, for example, have 4.27 calories in each gram of protein. The amount of protein in a weight of a food varies markedly. If a food is dry, like gluten flour, the percentage will be high, compared to lean meat which contains a lot of water in its weight.

Protein in Cereals (percentage by weight)

Cake or pastry flour	7.5
Gluten flour	41.4
Wheat flour (all-purpose white)	10.5
Whole-wheat flour	13.0
Cornmeal (whole-grain or nearly whole-grain)	9.2
Oatmeal (dry)	14.2
Rice (dry, uncooked)	7.0
Wheat, shredded (and other whole-wheat products)	9.9

Cheese is a good source of protein. It is also very high in fat, particularly saturated fat. If for some reason you must avoid too much fat in your diet, cheese is not a good choice for your protein. Remember, with the exception of cottage cheese, nearly 80 per cent of the calories in cheese are from fat and half these fat calories are saturated fat. Uncreamed cottage cheese, however, is an excellent source of protein (and calcium) and is a low-fat food. The protein in cheese, since it comes from milk, is a complete protein of high quality. It is valuable for both growth and maintenance.

Protein in Cheeses (percentage by weight)

Cheddar cheese	25.0
Cream cheese	8.0
Creamed cottage cheese	13.6
Uncreamed cottage cheese	17.0

With the exception of cottage cheese, to get enough protein in your diet from cheese alone you would need to eat an enormous number of calories. Only about a fourth of the calories in cheddar cheese is from protein and most of the rest are from fat.

Eggs are an excellent source of protein, and the proteins in eggs are complete proteins. You might expect this since the food in an egg is packaged by Mother Nature to provide the materials for growth of the developing chick. The only problem with eggs is the high content of cholesterol in the yolk and the relatively high fat content. Incidentally, by feeding the hens foods containing polyunsaturated fat, the fat content can be altered to contain less saturated fat and more unsaturated fat.

You can avoid the high-fat, high-cholesterol content in eggs and still enjoy them by using some of the new low-fat, low-cholesterol products now on the market for that purpose. Egg whites are nearly all protein and water and you can use unlimited quantities of them in your diet without affecting your cholesterol and fat intake.

Protein in Eggs (percentage by weight)

Whole egg	12.9
Egg white	10.9
Egg yolk	16.0

As a guide, a whole egg weighs about 50 grams (1¾ ounces); one egg white, 33 grams (1⅙ ounces); and one yolk, 17 grams (⁶⁄₁₀ ounce).

Milk is an excellent source of protein. Nature designed milk to support growth of the young, and its protein is excellent for growth. Whole milk is often classified as a high-protein food, but less than a fourth of its calories are from protein and half of its calories are from fat. It is better classified as a high-fat food. Moreover, a large portion of its fat is of the saturated type. If you want to limit the amount of fat in your diet, whole milk is not a good food choice. The dairy industry has remedied that problem, though, and you can get fortified skim milk which is essentially a fat-free food with a great deal of protein. You can also use nonfat dry milk powder in cooking as a good source of protein and calcium. I must caution you that you should not do without milk or a satisfactory milk substitute. In our diet, milk and milk products, such as uncreamed cottage cheese, are among our few good sources of calcium. In general I believe all adults should get at least a quart of milk a day or its equivalent in other milk products to meet the calcium needs of the body.

Individuals who cannot tolerate milk because of inability to digest the milk sugar, lactose, can use milk substitutes. These are made mostly from soybean products. You can find them in the baby-food department of most supermarkets. Be careful, though. Some artificial milks are made with coconut oil and so are high in saturated fat. Read the label critically. And since fermentation decreases the amount of lactose in milk, buttermilk and uncreamed cottage cheese may be tolerated better than milk.

Protein in Milk (percentage by weight)

Whole milk	3.5
Skim milk fortified with	
2 per cent nonfat milk solids	4.2
Buttermilk	3.6

As you see, there is actually more protein in fortified skim milk than there is in whole milk. Using whole milk as a guide, there is a gram of protein in an ounce of milk. Remember the old adage, "A pint's a pound the world around." It follows that a pint of milk, 16 ounces, contains about 16 grams of good protein, more if it's fortified skim milk, and a quart contains 32 grams of protein. If you use the metric system, a half liter of milk should contain a little more than 16 grams of protein. An 8-ounce cup or glass of milk then would provide 8 grams of protein for your diet.

You shouldn't think of bread as a rich source of protein unless it is made with gluten flour or by using a special recipe. You can add a number of egg whites to homemade bread and markedly increase its protein content. The protein in bread, otherwise, is from milk and wheat. What you get is a high-quality protein.

Protein in Bread (percentage by weight)

Enriched white bread	8.7
Whole-wheat bread	10.5
Biscuits and dinner rolls	7.4

Most of the vegetables do not contain much protein. The percentage of the calories as protein may be higher than you would expect, simply because a number of vegetables are low-calorie foods. The protein in vegetables is not as good as that found in animal products. That means you need to eat more of it to achieve the same effect. Legumes contain a lot of protein, but the protein in white or navy beans is incomplete and they are low in cystine. Some nutritionists place great emphasis on cystine. Cystine can be, and is, manufactured from the essential amino acid methionine. If the diet contains abundant amounts of methionine, and it should if it is a good diet, there should not be a cystine shortage. Even so, the mature bean seed protein is nearly complete and goes a long way in providing the protein requirements, particularly for maintenance. Peas also have incomplete proteins, also low in cystine. Soybeans, however, contain both complete and incomplete proteins. The combination means that soybeans in sufficient amounts could meet the body's protein needs, even for growth. This is why soybeans are an important staple in many cultures and in vegetarian diets.

Protein in Beans (percentage by weight)

Beans, white or navy, mature seeds, raw	22.3
cooked	7.8
Lima beans, mature seeds, raw	20.4
immature seeds, raw	8.4
Peas, green, raw	6.3
mature, raw	24.1
Soybeans, mature, raw	34.1
immature, raw	10.9

Mushrooms would hardly constitute a major portion of many people's diet. But a high percentage of their calories are from protein, as a vegetarian friend pointed out to me. Raw mushrooms are 2.7 per cent protein by weight (2.7 grams per 100 grams of mushrooms). Canned mushrooms are only 1.9 per cent protein by weight. Nevertheless, this represents a fourth to a third of the total calories in mushrooms. As a standard of comparison, less than one-fourth of the total calories in whole milk are protein.

Fruits, berries, and melons have small amounts of protein, so small that you might as well forget about them as a protein source. Moreover, the protein is not very digestible. The only exception to this statement is the dried fruits. If you eat raisins or dried prunes, the amount of protein by weight is markedly increased because the water has been removed.

The protein from animal muscles resembles the protein in our muscle. Myosin is present in all of them. Remember that the more nearly a protein resembles the protein in our body, the more completely and readily it will be used.

Fish is an excellent protein source. Because it contains a lot of water it is also a low-calorie food. It is interesting to note that, despite certain folklore concepts about eating oysters to increase sexual powers, they are lower in protein than most shellfish and fish.

Protein in Seafood (percentage by weight)

Codfish, raw	17.6
Flounder, raw	16.7
cooked, baked	30.0
Lobster, Northern, raw	16.9
Oysters, raw	9.5
Red Snapper, raw	19.8
Shrimp, raw	18.1

As with other foods listed, these values apply only to the edible part. In the case of fish, this means the actual flesh to be eaten, without bones.

Poultry—chicken or turkey—is an excellent choice for a protein source. It contains complete protein. There is some variation in the protein content of various pieces and whether you are using a frying chicken or a roaster. But as a satisfactory guide, about 20 per cent of the edible flesh is protein. When it is cooked, because of water loss about 28 per cent of the weight of the edible part is protein. The white meat contains a slightly higher percentage of protein, and turkey contains a little more protein than chicken. The protein in beef is much like that in our muscles. The only problem in using beef as a protein source is that beef fat is high in saturated fat and low in polyunsaturated fat. Even so, if you use lean cuts and are careful in preparing it, you can use beef on a relatively low-fat diet. But you should not use beef to the exclusion of fish and poultry. The amount of protein in the various cuts listed below will give you a general idea how much protein you get in beef. The values are for the edible part only:

Protein in Beef (edible part only) (percentage by weight)

Entire chuck	
total edible, raw	18.7
cooked	26.0
separable lean, raw	21.3
separable lean, cooked	30.0
T-Bone steak	
choice, raw	14.7
choice, broiled	19.5
choice, separable lean, raw	21.2
choice, separable lean, broiled	30.4
good, raw	15.4
good, broiled	20.6
good, separable lean, raw	21.5
good, separable lean, broiled	31.1
Round steak	
choice, raw, total	20.2
broiled	28.6
separable lean, raw	21.6
broiled	31.3

Veal is nearly the same as beef in terms of protein content.

The amount of protein in pork is particularly dependent on how much of the weight is fat. A very fatty piece, for example cured bacon, will have a considerably lower percentage of protein content than lean ham. As a guide to the protein content in pork the following values for a composite of trimmed lean cuts (ham, loin, shoulder, spare ribs) from a medium-fat-class carcass are suitable:

Protein in Pork (percentage by weight)

Total edible, raw	15.7
cooked	22.6
Separable lean	19.1
cooked	28.0

Lamb is still another source of excellent protein, but, like the other mammal meats, you must limit your intake if you want to avoid saturated fat. The composite cuts trimmed to retail level from a choice lamb contain 16.5 per cent protein.

Cold cuts contain meat protein, so it is good protein, but there will be less of it. Much of the food value in cold cuts is from fat. As much as 80 per cent of the calories in salami, bologna, and similar meats are from fat. Only about 12 per cent of the weight of bologna and frankfurters is protein.

Gelatin should be considered here. It is an animal product derived from the connective tissue, including tendons, that holds us together. If you save the drippings from a roast, they gel as they cool. It is the gelatin protein that does this. Fish, poultry, and mammal meat all contain this protein. It is not considered a high-quality protein, but it is rich in lysine. It is a valuable protein to combine with cereals to meet the amino-acid requirements. It is a poor protein only because it doesn't contain a lot of the essential amino acids. It is useful to provide enough of the total amount of protein your body needs. Dry gelatin is almost pure protein—85.6 per cent by weight.

Desserts can be a source of protein, but most of them are not. Clearly, gelatin desserts contain protein. Any dessert that uses a lot of milk will add to your protein intake. Custard is a good example. Desserts are not necessarily all bad—as some would have you believe. The biggest problem is that many of them contain too much fat and too much carbohydrate. Both may be calories without any valuable quantities of protein, vitamins, or minerals. This can be overcome in part by making some desserts using dry skim-milk powder or fortified skim milk. You can also add to the protein intake by adding egg whites to pies, cakes, cookies, and puddings. If you want to use a lot of egg whites you can build up the protein content of a dessert rather fast. Some protein powders can also be used as additives to a dessert to increase the protein content. You can also use polyunsaturated oil in place of saturated fats in making the dessert. In general, then, the protein content of a dessert depends entirely on how it is made.

The nut group contains protein, but nuts are also high in fat.

Protein in Nuts (percentage by weight)

Almonds	18.6
Peanuts	26.0
Pecans	9.2
Walnuts, black	20.5
Walnuts, Persian or English	14.8

Now you should be in a position to formulate a simple menu that provides all the protein your body needs. Remember, for an adult a goal of 70 grams of protein a day is adequate. If you are pregnant or engaged in a body-building program, you may need more. I usually recommend that everyone get a quart of milk a day—and I hope it will be fortified skim milk. You can count on at least 32 grams of protein a day this way. Also you should have eight ounces (230 grams) of either meat, fish, or poultry (edible part, raw). You can estimate that the edible raw portion of fish, mammal meat, and poultry will contain 17.5 per cent protein (5 grams in each ounce). So 8 ounces (230 grams) will provide 40 grams of protein. All these foods contain complete proteins so your body will be getting all the essential amino acids. Of course, you can use uncreamed cottage cheese, or you can use milk or milk powder in cooking. The additional protein will provide a good safeguard. If you can't use meat, I'd recommend using a lot of soybean products as a substitute. You would need nearly 4 ounces (115 grams) of mature seeds to provide 40 grams of protein. You could also increase your milk or milk-product intake or increase the egg whites in your diet. As you see, you can meet your protein requirements very easily and still not eat a high-fat, high-saturated-fat diet. Just use low-fat dairy products and rotate your meat dish among mammal meat, fish, and poultry.

Now, about those protein powders and tablets. Should you use them? That depends. If you have a well-balanced diet with enough protein and sufficient quantities of all the essential amino acids, there is no need to take additional protein either as powder or as tablets. That excess protein is just like excess shingles for a house: you could burn them for fuel in the house. The body does that with the excess protein from powders and tablets and uses them for energy (calories) or stores their energy in the form of fat. The energy in protein is no better than the energy in carbohydrates or fats.

Proteins may not be as desirable a source of energy as carbohydrates or fat if your work requires heavy exertion. Why? Because too much of the energy from protein breakdown is dissipated as heat energy rather than being available for ATP and physical work. That has two disadvantages, the loss of available energy and the tendency to overheat the body. A buildup of body heat during exertion detracts from your maximum ability. This feature of proteins is a result of their specific dynamic action, which I'll discuss later.

If you are not getting all your protein requirements from your diet, then protein supplements are useful. Let's say you can't tolerate milk. That is a major loss of diet protein, and unless you eat a lot of animal food items, you may not get enough protein. In this case an additional source of protein would be helpful. What about the teenager who likes sweets, soft drinks, cold cuts, and hot dogs but won't touch milk, meat, or eggs? You could be sneaky and serve him some high-protein desserts and high-protein homemade bread, made by putting milk, eggs, and particularly egg whites into them. Or you could encourage him to use the protein supplements.

There are people with a host of digestive problems that interfere with absorption from the intestine. Some of these people also profit from adding protein supplements to their diet. As I mentioned, gelatin can help some in this regard if there is enough complete protein in the diet. Then there are the older people and those who live alone who do not eat an adequate diet. This is probably the largest group of people who need protein supplements. You might get an eighty-year-old woman who likes only sweets to drink a mixture of protein powder, tastefully sweetened and flavored, but she may refuse to eat meat.

Still another large group who can profit from using protein supplements are those who must seriously decrease the fat intake in their diet. I have in mind those with a very high cholesterol level or heart disease. The protein supplements can provide a good source of proteins when meat dishes, eggs, and milk are curtailed. Of course, such a person could use low-fat fish, fortified skim milk, and other protein foods.

Some people must strictly limit their salt intake. If the limitation is severe, there will have to be a limitation on milk, meats, fish, poultry, and many of the foods that provide complete protein because all these foods contain salt. Soybean products are useful here. But these people can also use protein supplements to keep up their protein intake while limiting salt.

With the growing world-wide food problem, serious thought should be given to making protein supplements more readily available. They can be made fairly easily, and in large quantities should be quite cheap. Most of the current commercially available protein powders and protein supplements are grossly overpriced, at many times the cost of production.

11

HOW YOU USE PROTEINS

After you eat all those proteins how does the body process them? They are all treated much alike. The process begins in the stomach. The stomach wall pours out its hydrochloric acid and the enzyme pepsin. The acid digestive juice goes to work on the proteins, breaking them down into polypeptides, the smaller units of amino acids. It is important to understand this because it explains in part why you can't simply swallow certain foods and expect them to appear unaltered in the bloodstream. Any food that is a protein begins its breakdown in the stomach. This is why insulin is not given by mouth to treat diabetics. Remember insulin is a protein made from fifty-one amino-acid units. Just as soon as these arrive in the stomach they are rapidly torn down into smaller clusters of amino acids, the polypeptides.

Proteins tend to remain in the stomach longer than carbohydrates but not as long as fats. When liquefied, the proteins, along with the other food nutrients, are squirted into the duodenum, the first part of the small intestine. Once in the small intestine the polypeptides are exposed to the pancreatic juice. It contains two enzymes that attack the polypeptide groups, which for simplicity here we will call the trypsin enzymes. Incidentally, trypsin comes from the cleavage of a parent enzyme, called trypsinogen, which contains 229 amino-acid units. The pancreatic enzymes break the polypeptides into still smaller units called peptides.

The smaller peptide units are still not ready for the bloodstream. The intestinal wall pours out still other enzymes called peptidases. These split the peptides down into the simple amino acids. Now protein in your food can be absorbed. As you see, the stomach, the pancreas, and even the small intestine pour out enzymes that must act on proteins to prepare them for absorption. When the amino-acid units are finally ready for absorption, it doesn't matter whether the amino acid came from insulin, beefsteak, milk, soybeans, or whatever. At the most there would be twenty-five different types of amino acids and any one amino acid such as glycine is glycine regardless of its source. It's the same as saying a brick is a brick regardless of which house it came from.

You may be surprised to know that the protein in your food is only part of the protein absorbed from the intestine into your bloodstream. Remember that the cells lining the small intestine flake off regularly at the rate of a half pound a day. Then there are all those proteins in the secretions from the salivary glands, pepsin, pancreatic juice, and enzymes composed of proteins. In all, there are about 150 grams of protein from the secretions and, by a conservative estimate, 25 to 30 grams in discarded cells a day. The protein from your own body, then, that ends up in the intestine each day totals about 150 to 180 grams. This perfectly good protein is mixed with your food protein into a common pool of protein parts or polypeptides, peptides, and finally amino acids.

The mixed pool of amino acids from your body and from your food is rapidly absorbed through the intestinal wall into the bloodstream. The transport of amino acids again takes energy. Everywhere you turn you will find the body uses energy to move elements and compounds through cells in the body. The body uses an enormous amount of energy each day just in doing its own thing, before you even consider physical activity and the energy balance.

The amino acids from your body and those in your food are equal in the amino-acid marketplace in your body. Either can be used to build new cells or form new protein for more secretions. They are just like a dollar bill—its purchasing power is not affected by whether it is old or new. Our body is very thrifty and it recycles many of its own products rather than waste them. Once the amino acids are in the blood they are quickly removed, mostly by the liver.

Most of the newly arrived amino acids are trapped in the liver for their initial preparation for use. The liver strips off the amino unit of one nitrogen and two hydrogen blocks, leaving the amino acid much like a fatty acid or glucose-type product. The process is called deamination. Since about 90 per cent of this type of activity occurs in the liver, for practical purposes you can consider deamination a function of the liver.

The next problem is to get rid of the amino group. If it is not needed to form new amino acids and the remainder of the amino acid is to be used for energy, the amino group is converted to urea. This is the substance that gives urine its name. Urea is nothing more than two units of amino groups hooked together with a unit of carbon dioxide. You can think of it as a combination of blocks like Figure 27.

Let's use the amino acid alanine to see how deamination works.

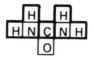

Fig. 27. A simplified block diagram
of urea from two amino (NHH)
units from amino acids.

Alanine is a simple three-carbon-chain amino acid. Deamination in this
case uses the coenzyme NAD and a unit of water. The NAD picks up
two hydrogen blocks from the water. Alanine picks up the oxygen from
the water as it gives up a nitrogen block and three hydrogen blocks, or
simple ammonia (see Figure 28).

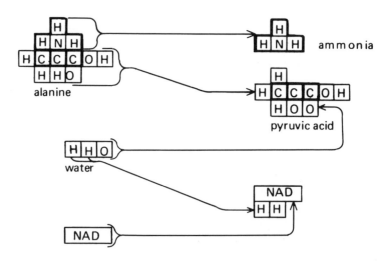

Fig. 28. Converting the amino acid alanine to pyruvic acid by stripping off the amino group.

Just as it does in so many other situations, NAD passes its hydrogen
along the respiratory chain to react with oxygen and form water. As
always, this process yields energy and stores it as ATP. Through a sec-

ond chain of reactions the ammonia is combined with carbon dioxide to form urea. By stripping off the ammonia and giving the carbon skeleton a unit of oxygen, it becomes a familiar unit of pyruvic acid. And there you have it, an amino acid converted to a carbon unit in the chain of glucose metabolism. The pyruvic acid formed this way is no different from pyruvic acid formed from glucose. It can continue down the metabolic route to be broken apart and release energy or it can go back up the chain to form blood glucose. Of course it can also take the path from acetic acid to be converted to fat.

Urea is formed exclusively in the liver. It is released into the bloodstream and filtered out by our kidneys. Not really a toxin, it's harmless unless a person has serious kidney failure and the amount retained in the blood becomes very high.

Many of the amino acids can be stripped of their ammonia and converted to one of the carbon skeletons that is part of the glucose metabolic process. These amino acids are called glucogenic (*gluco* for glucose, *genic* for genesis or birth).

Glucogenic Amino Acids

Alanine	Hydroxyproline
Arginine	Ornithine
Aspartic Acid	Proline
Cysteine	Serine
Cystine	Threonine
Glutamic Acid	Valine
Glycine	

Other amino acids which are stripped of their ammonia are converted to acetic acid or the ketone acetoacetic acid. They can form ketone bodies and are known as the ketogenic amino acids. These can be converted directly to fat through the formation of active acetate. Of course the glucogenic amino acids can also be converted to fat once they enter the glucose metabolic processing system.

Ketogenic Amino Acids

Isoleucine	Phenylalanine
Leucine	Tyrosine

The amino acids norleucine, methionine, lysine, and histidine are not converted to either glucose or ketones. Look at the flow diagram to see how the glucogenic and ketogenic amino acids fit into the metabolic system. As a general guide, a mixed sample of protein with a variety of amino acids produces 58 grams of glucose in the body.

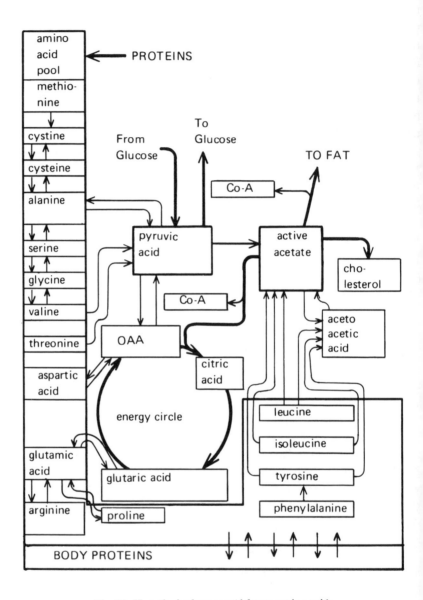

Fig. 29. How the body uses and forms amino acids.

Almost all the amino acids that come to the liver are deaminated. The spare amino group stripped off is then used to form new amino acids. Transferring the amino group to another carbon skeleton is called transamination. Here's how it works: A unit of glutamic acid arrives in the liver and is quickly stripped of its ammonia. Now if there is some pyruvic acid around, and there will be, the ammonia is simply hooked on to the pyruvic acid to form the new amino acid, alanine. In the process, glutamic acid has been converted to a carbon skeleton in the glucose metabolic chain (alpha ketoglutaric acid of the citric-acid cycle) of the energy circle common to all foods converted to energy. In a similar way all manner of new amino acids can be formed except the essential amino acids, which must be supplied by the food.

Although deamination occurs almost exclusively in the liver, transamination is a function of cells in general. This process can occur anywhere. The cells can take ammonia from other compounds (commonly left over from deamination) to use in transamination.

The deamination and transamination of the carbon chains, the essential amino acids in the food you eat, and the breakdown of body protein provide the body with an "amino acid pool." The pool contains the free amino acids in the cells available for building. This pool is constantly being replenished with amino acids from food and from the breakdown of protein within the body. There is a fairly constant turnover of the amino acids in the tissues, probably the result of the continual loss of cells and their replacement. A good example here is the constant turnover of the red blood cells. This involves constant destruction and regeneration of cells. The vital proteins in the blood, such as globulin and albumin, are constantly being torn down and rebuilt. Within tissue cells of organs the most rapid turnover is of the cells of the liver, kidneys, and intestinal tract.

As amino acids are made available from the breakdown of tissue protein, the protein is rebuilt. This means that even though nitrogen is released when the amino acids are deaminated, an equal amount of nitrogen in the amino group is used in the rebuilding process. As long as the rebuilding process matches the tearing-down process, a constant amount of nitrogen will be retained in the body. In these circumstances the amino acids in your food aren't so necessary, except for exchange to provide essential amino acids. The amino group torn off will be converted to urea and eliminated by the kidneys. Some nitrogen is also eliminated with the food residue. When your body is rebuilding at the same rate of breakdown, you will eliminate the same amount of nitrogen from the kidneys and bowel as you take in. This state is spoken of as *nitrogen balance.*

If for any reason tissue breakdown is faster than tissue building, you will be losing more nitrogen than you get in your food. This is called *negative nitrogen balance.* This occurs in starvation when the body proteins are processed for energy and the amino group stripped off is a waste product. A negative nitrogen balance is an indication of a gradual break-down of important body tissues.

During growth, such as occurs in an active teenager, there will be more new tissue formed than is breaking down. In this case a good bit of the nitrogen in the proteins in the diet will be retained by the body as it uses the amino acids in the pool to build new structures. Less nitrogen will be eliminated than taken in. This is spoken of as a *positive nitrogen balance*. A positive nitrogen balance is an indication of growth of new muscles and cells and formation of protein secretions (not fat cells or storage).

The grand scheme of protein metabolism is to add amino acids to the mixture of those from our own bodies to form a pool. When the total amount of amino acids is more than is needed for building, the leftover amino acids are stripped and the carbon skeleton is used for energy or stored as fat. When you are in balance the amount stripped off and eliminated should equal the amount in your diet.

Carbohydrates and fat serve as protein-sparing sources of energy. The body must have a minimal amount of energy to carry on its basic cell functions. It is sometimes called the basal metabolism. This is where all that hidden energy goes that we don't use for physical activity. The energy needs can easily be met by the energy locked in the carbohydrates and fat. If they are not present in the diet, the body will use protein for energy. Any time amino acids are stripped of the amino group and used for energy, they are no longer available for building. By sparing the amino acids from being broken down and stripped of their energy, the glucose and fatty acids allow them to be available for the building pro-cess. Many patients are given glucose in water by vein when they can't eat to provide them an energy source and spare the body protein from being used for this purpose.

The sparing action of carbohydrates is not entirely shared by fat. A diet of fat alone will not spare the proteins, and the body tissues will begin to break down, creating a negative nitrogen balance. If half of the calories are carbohydrate, and enough fats and carbohydrates are pro-vided, they will spare the body protein. It has been stated that even a diet of protein and fat alone will not spare the body protein. The validity of this observation is not entirely evident. It has been suggested that the sugars are essential in some chemical step between the breakdown of amino acids and their formation, perhaps by transamination. In any case, to spare the body protein it's a good idea to have some carbohydrate in the diet.

As an example of the importance of this sparing action, if there is no pyruvic acid present or if there is not enough of it, it might be difficult to form a whole group of amino acids that depends on adding an amino group to pyruvic acid. Let's say that an amino acid was deaminated in the liver and the carbon skeletons were used for energy. The amino group could be transferred to pyruvic acid to form alanine, but if you are short on pyruvic acid because you don't have any carbohydrate in the diet, this will not occur so readily. In this way a shortage of carbohydrate could affect the body's ability to form new protein.

Another curious aspect of protein metabolism that is poorly understood is the basis for a lot of people thinking you lose weight from eating protein. The statement is often made that proteins burn other calories. This refers to a phenomenon called the specific dynamic action of protein. Don't let that term scare you. The concept is really simple. A lot of the energy in amino acids is not made available either for the cell work of moving chemicals or as physical work. It is lost as heat. From laboratory studies you would expect to have four calories in a gram of a certain protein; yet in the body it yields far less for body processes because part of the calories are converted to heat rather than being used to form ATP units.

It is not clear why the heat is produced, but it is thought to be released when the bonds that connect the amino group to the carbon skeleton are broken. This would account for heat's unique relation to proteins. Furthermore, the heat is generated chiefly in the liver, where almost all of the deamination occurs. This has some practical aspects. When you are planning the amount of calories you need, it is quite true that you will need more calories if a major portion of the food comes from protein than you would if it came from carbohydrates. This demonstrates that proteins are not an efficient food for energy despite their importance as building materials. Your body can use both carbohydrates and fat more efficiently for energy. It also means that if you are concerned about excess body heat, protein is a poor choice for energy. A heavy laborer, particularly in a hot climate, will do better getting his energy from carbohydrates and fat and limiting the protein in the diet to provide building material. To avoid additional body heat the proteins could be eaten in that part of the day when labor is not being performed. Before the days of air conditioning, many people knew they would feel better in the hot summer months if they ate more fruits, vegetables, and salads and less meat. When you consider the effects of protein on body heat production, you can understand why they were right.

The very substances of life itself are related to protein metabolism. These substances are the fascinating nucleic acids, DNA and RNA.

DNA, which has become well known in recent years, is the same thing as the genes that pass on our hereditary traits. They determine the characteristics of our cells, the color of our hair and eyes, and all of our body features. And we have a complete set of DNA building instructions for the entire body in each of our cells. The instructions are in the first-formed cell from the union of the sperm and the ovum. Each new cell gets its own copy of the building plan. RNA is the processing line in the ribosomes of the cell plasma around the nucleus. It processes all these amino acids to form new proteins.

Let's think of insulin for a minute. It is a complex protein. All fifty-one amino-acid units are hooked together to form the insulin unit by an assembly-line technique on a strip of RNA.

You may be surprised to know that DNA and RNA are closely related to gout. How your DNA and RNA are made has a lot more to do with whether you will have gout than all of the food you eat. Those pictures you have seen of the fat man with gout, his foot resting on a stool with a red swollen toe exposed, a glass of wine in one hand and a leg of lamb in the other, are poor representations of the facts. Gout is caused by too much uric acid in the body, and too much uric acid is usually caused by DNA and RNA production.

Uric acid is a side product of purine. You have no doubt heard some reference to purine-free diets. Purine is not protein, though it is made of three amino acids: glutamic acid, glycine, and aspartic acid. Its structure is complicated in the way the blocks are hooked together, but it is made of simple carbon, hydrogen, nitrogen, and oxygen blocks. It contains five nitrogen blocks, a good deal more than you find in a single amino acid, but not necessarily more than you find in most proteins. The purines are often called purine bases. There are only two, adenine and guanine.

Adenine is no stranger to you. It combines with a sugar (ribose) and three phosphate units to form adenosine triphosphate or our energy shuttle, ATP. You can see how vital it is to the body's functions. Guanine is very similar to adenine. In the process of forming the purine bases the cell may manufacture uric acid, a closely related compound. Incidentally, one step on the way is the formation of xanthine, which is considered a drug. Caffeine in coffee is a drug of the xanthine group. It is a powerful brain stimulant. Perhaps the xanthine affects mental alertness in a manner similar to that of caffeine. This is interesting since many successful active people have had gout, among them Leonardo da Vinci, Ben Franklin, Frederick the Great, and many kings. Gout was once designated the disease of kings and the king of diseases.

Most cases of elevated uric acid are caused by overproduction of uric acid in the cells. An excessive breakdown of tissue with their nucleic acids, as can occur in starvation or leukemia, can also produce excessive amounts of uric acid. The amount of uric acid can be increased by failure of the kidneys to eliminate sufficient amounts. To a limited extent the diet can also be a contributing factor.

Since DNA and RNA are nucleic acids, they are found in large amounts in the nuclei of cells. It was early recognized that certain foods were rich in purines. These were the foods that contained cells with many nuclei, primarily the organ meats—liver, kidney, pancreas. Since there are bound to be many nuclei in all meat foods, a purine-free diet was obviously one using milk, vegetables, cereals, and fruit. Milk contains no cellular elements and is definitely free of purine. This observation provides the basis for an interesting experiment. Even when a calf is fed nothing but milk it produces a lot of uric acid. It is clear then that the growing calf on a purine-free diet is manufacturing its own purines and hence uric acid.

Diet is important in gout. The most important consideration is usually to limit calories to prevent or eliminate obesity. If obesity is to be eliminated it should be done slowly to avoid a rapid tissue destruction which can increase the uric acid and precipitate an attack of gout. As you'll see later, in crash diet programs part of the weight loss is from the breakdown of body protein, mostly muscle tissue. The gout patient's diet should be regulated to provide a good quality diet and to avoid obesity and problems related to atherosclerosis and heart disease. The idea of eliminating all purine sources has more or less been dropped. We know that even on a strict no-purine diet you can lower the amount of uric acid in the blood only a small amount. Medicines are usually needed to lower it to the proper levels. One of the new medicines, allopurinol (Zyloprim), acts by preventing the cell from forming uric acid while it is forming new purine bases. Other medicines act by helping to increase the elimination of uric acid through the kidneys.

A group of compounds closely related to purines are the pyrimidine bases. These contain three nitrogen building blocks and are also made from amino acids. The three pyrimidine bases are cytosine, uracil, and thymine. They do not form uric acid. The purine bases and pyrimidine bases are used in the formation of DNA and RNA. The process is complex but it can be simplified by a simple diagram. A base—for example, adenine—is hooked on to the sugar unit and the sugar unit is hooked to the phosphate unit. A single strand of blocks like this is RNA (Figure 30). Notice that the successive units of sugar, phosphate, sugar, phosphate, and so on form a running ribbon of chemical compounds. The base units stick up like teeth.

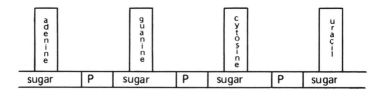

Fig. 30. A strip of RNA.

The unattached end of the base unit (adenosine or other) can connect to another base unit from a second strand of RNA. The result is a double strand, or DNA. The manner of hooking together the variety of bases of purines and pyrimidines provides the chemical sequence that determines what we are and the ability of our cells to replace themselves. They are the basis of life and its repetitive process, and they can all be built from the food you eat. The original blueprint in your body when the egg was fertilized determines how all the basic building blocks in your food are going to be arranged to produce you and to maintain you for your life span.

12

GETTING ENERGY FROM ALCOHOL

Have you heard that alcoholic beverages don't contain calories? Don't you believe it. In fact, alcohol is very much like a fatty acid and contains almost as many calories (7 calories per gram). The alcohol in drinking beverages is ethyl alcohol, a simple two-carbon block unit saturated with hydrogen. It could qualify as a two-carbon bit sliced from a fatty acid chain. Figure 31 is a simple block diagram of ethyl alcohol.

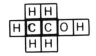

Fig. 31. A simplified block diagram of ethyl alcohol.

Alcohol is a common source of calories in many people's diet. About 68 per cent of all Americans drink alcohol and about 12 per cent are heavy drinkers. That means a drink almost every day and on occasions five or more cocktails. Americans don't have a monopoly on alcohol. The use of alcohol goes back before Biblical times. Man had to content himself with simple fermented beverages, however, that were relatively weak in alcoholic content but nevertheless effective. The Arabs introduced the distilling process which led to whiskey.

Just to show you how wrong sages can be, the wise men of the age thought it was the "elixir of life" and that is why it is called whiskey, an old Gaelic word meaning "water of life." We know now that it actually shortens life. Alcoholism is a world-wide problem. In the United States it is the third most common cause of death, just behind circulatory disease and cancer. The toll in human suffering caused by alcohol dwarfs the problems caused by the high death rate from alcohol.

Do you have any idea how much alcohol is in your drinks and what the body does with the alcohol? If so, you are better informed than most people. You need to know since this is a key factor in how your body responds to drinking. Most whiskey, gin, and similar beverages are labeled in proof. You need to know how much alcohol there is in an ounce (about 29 milliliters).

Amount of Spirits Yielding a Half Ounce of Alcohol

80 proof	1.5 ounces
86 proof	1.4
90 proof	1.3
94 proof	1.25
100 proof	1.2

Since cocktails are usually mixed by the jigger, let's translate those numbers into what really happens. A jigger by definition is supposed to contain 1.5 ounces. The jigger in common use, however, really contains only 1.0 to 1.25 ounces. To limit the amount of alcohol in your cocktail to not more than a half ounce, you should use only one jigger of alcoholic beverage, using the common jigger of 1.0 to 1.25 ounces. That way, even if you use 100-proof spirits you won't greatly exceed a half ounce of alcohol.

A 12-ounce can of beer (4.5 per cent alcohol by volume, 3.6 per cent by weight) contains 0.43 ounces of alcohol. Table wines (12.2 per cent alcohol by volume and 9.9 per cent by weight) are fairly strong. Four or 5 ounces will provide about a half ounce of alcohol. Dessert wines such as sherry and port are even stronger (18.9 per cent alcohol by volume and 15.3 per cent by weight). You will need to go easy on them if you want to avoid ingesting excess amounts of alcohol. It was indeed fortunate that such wines were planned for after the meal, slowing the absorption of alcohol into the blood.

In general, then, cocktails made with one jigger of beverage, a 12-ounce can of beer, 4 or 5 ounces of table wine, and less of dessert wine, are about equal in alcohol content.

A big factor in determining how much alcohol gets into the blood, and how soon, is its absorption from the stomach and small intestine. Alcohol is very much like water in that it needs no processing to be absorbed.

Proteins, fats, and carbohydrates must all be broken down by enzymes before they can be absorbed, but not alcohol. Some of it can be absorbed from the stomach, but this is a slow process. As soon as it reaches the small intestine it is absorbed extremely rapidly. Remember that over a fourth of the water you drink is absorbed from the small intestine within a minute. Within ten minutes at the most all the alcohol that arrives in your small intestine will be absorbed into the blood. This means that the main factor determining how rapidly the alcohol you drink will be in your blood is how long it takes it to get through the stomach.

Obviously there is a sound basis for the common idea that if you want to avoid getting drunk you should not drink on an empty stomach. Liquids do tend to spread out around the solid food mass in the stomach, but, even so, the emptying process is delayed, and usually long enough for much of the alcohol to be absorbed into the food mass and diluted. Then the rate at which the alcohol will be emptied into the intestine and absorbed directly into the blood will depend entirely on how fast that mass of food is liquefied and emptied from the stomach. Remember, fatty foods empty slowly, and this is the basis for the observation that drinking cream or eating any fatty food before a drinking bout will increase one's tolerance for alcohol. Don't be misled—all that alcohol in the stomach is eventually emptied into the intestine and then processed. The full stomach just prolongs the absorption time required to do the job. This is important, though, because it limits the amount of alcohol that arrives in the blood at one time.

When the stomach is still full of food and a person is getting drunk, vomiting serves a protective function. It prevents what alcohol remains in the stomach from being added to a bad situation. Once the alcohol is in the bloodstream, it is processed by your metabolic machinery at a constant rate. You can't speed up the process. Drinking coffee and all manner of attempted treatments won't help. The average-sized adult will break down about 10 milliliters (one-third of an ounce) of alcohol an hour. Given this constant rate of using the alcohol, you can see that the concentration of alcohol in the blood is almost entirely dependent on how fast it is absorbed.

The two-carbon alcohol unit is converted by special enzymes, and some intermediate steps, to active acetate (acetyl–Co-A). It is now in the metabolic cycle. The acetate unit can be split from the Co-A and, in the presence of oxygen, be put through the energy circle to yield energy, or it can take the fat path for fat formation. It can be used to form ketone bodies, or even to make cholesterol. Figure 32 is a simplified diagram of the processing line for alcohol.

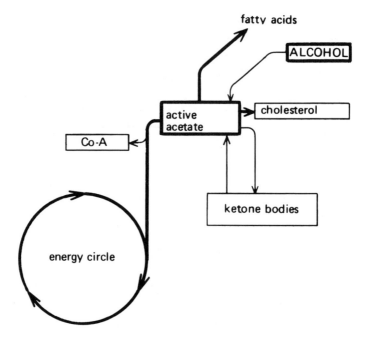

Fig. 32. Processing alcohol.

Although alcohol has many effects on the body, its relation to the function and performance of the brain is of particular importance. This depends entirely on how much alcohol there is in the blood. For this reason blood alcohol levels are used as an index of sobriety and, particularly, to determine whether it is safe for a person to drive.

In many parts of the United States if the blood alcohol is over .10 per cent the individual is said to be legally drunk. This does not mean that any one person will be functioning at his best even at blood alcohol levels lower than this.

Knowing how much alcohol there is in drinks, how it is absorbed, and how slowly it is broken down in the body, you can formulate some rules to stay within the .10 per cent blood level. Remember, you can't break down more than a third of an ounce (10 milliliters) of alcohol an hour. If you are going to have one drink, with one jigger of spirits, drink it

Effects of Different Concentrations of Alcohol in the Blood

Less than 0.05 per cent	Still sober
.05 to .10	Variable (may show some effects of alcohol)
.10 to .15	Under the influence, garrulous, euphoric, clumsy
.15 to .20	Obvious evidence of intoxication
.20 to .25	Stumbling and falling
.25 to .30	Drowsy and sleepy
.30 to .40	Stupor
.40 to .60	Coma and in the state of general anesthesia
over .60	Usually fatal

slowly over an hour's time if you plan to drive. Don't gulp the last part of it.

If you are going to have more than one drink use the following rules:

1. Drink no more than one-half ounce of alcohol each hour (the amount in one cocktail, one can of beer, or 5 ounces of table wine).
2. Drink no more than four drinks in succession at this rate of one an hour.
3. Wait one hour after the last drink before driving.

During the four hours' drinking time, with these rules, you will have drunk 2 ounces of alcohol. Assuming the worst, that it is on a nearly empty stomach, it would all be absorbed almost immediately. Your body would break down one-third ounce an hour, or a total of one and one-third ounces of alcohol. That leaves two-thirds of an ounce unaccounted for. By waiting an hour after the last drink, you allow the amount to get down to one-third ounce.

If your stomach was totally empty to begin with, and remains so through such a drinking bout, you will have a significantly high blood alcohol level. Assuming you do eat something, or ate something before, the absorption will be prolonged and the likelihood is that your blood alcohol will be down to the .10 per cent level, if you only have one drink an hour for four hours. If you have not eaten anything before or during drinking, you should limit your intake to three drinks, each containing no more than a half ounce of alcohol. Then you should wait an hour before driving or consume your three drinks over a four-hour period.

The alcohol in the bloodstream is absorbed directly into the cells. It tends to dry them out and coagulate the vital protein. In short, alcohol damages cells. Liver cell damage is so common that permanent damage and scarring of the liver can occur. Scarring of the liver is called cirrhosis. Incidentally, in defense of all those people with cirrhosis of the liver who do not have a drinking habit, it can be caused by a lot of other things too. This includes heart failure, poor nutrition, complications of gallstone problems, and various infections of the liver.

Evidence supports the idea that cell damage from drinking alcohol is not from a lack of proteins or vitamins in the diet. This has been hotly debated. The damage is a direct result of the alcohol itself. Bits of muscle tissue examined under a powerful electron microscope show cell damage when large quantities of alcohol were regularly consumed. This occurs even when the diet is quite adequate. The muscle fibers damaged can include the heart muscle. Individuals consuming large amounts of alcohol regularly can damage their heart muscle sufficiently to induce serious heart failure with retention of water causing shortness of breath and swellings. The condition is usually reversible when the alcohol consumption is stopped. The marvelous regenerative powers of our body simply replace the damaged tissue with new tissue.

The brain is seriously affected by alcohol. Some studies on mice have shown that amounts of alcohol equivalent to the amount consumed by many executives results in a failure to learn. This would suggest that the individual who wants to retain his learning capacity—which is desirable if he expects to have increased responsibility—should watch his drinking habits.

There is evidence that alcohol decreases the delivery of oxygen to the cells. You can guess at once what that means to the metabolic process. The problem results from "sludging," a phenomenon described by Dr. Melvin H. Knisely, a renowned physiologist. The process is simple: the red blood cells that normally glide smoothly past each other start clumping together. These small clumps can plug up the small vessels that feed blood and oxygen to the cells. You can even see this clumping effect in the small arteries in the back of the eye by looking directly into the eye of a person after he has been drinking. The more you drink the more vessels are plugged with clumped red blood cells. This may be a factor in the brain damage so often present in persons who have had a drinking habit over a period of time.

Any decrease in oxygen delivery caused by alcohol will affect the cell's ability to carry out aerobic metabolism releasing energy. Here then is a possible explanation for the tendency of alcoholics to get fat. Since alcohol is converted to active acetate you have all those two-carbon units ready to be processed. Because of the decreased amount of oxygen present they can take the fat path and be linked together to form fat. This way they are processed but don't provide any immediate energy. This may be the basis for the observation that the individual with a drinking problem tends to develop "whiskey fat." At the same time the alcohol is producing fat, it sops up energy, or at least uses that released in the original conversion of alcohol to active acetate. So the person is tired even though he may be consuming quite a large number of calories.

13

PUTTING YOUR ENERGY SYSTEM TOGETHER

By now you should have a pretty good idea what your body does with food. It might help you, though, to put it all together. This simple diagram shows the main things that happen to food. Although there are a lot of detailed steps, for most purposes you can summarize what happens into five very important statements. You should look at each of these statements and Figure 33 to make sure you understand them. These five basic principles will give you a working concept of what happens to your food.

1. All food, whether it is carbohydrates, fat, protein, or even alcohol, can be converted to fat, cholesterol, or energy. This is what happens to most of the food adults eat. If you eat more than you use for energy, it becomes fat and cholesterol. If you don't eat enough, you don't have enough energy.
2. The breakdown of food protein and body protein provides a mixture of amino acids called the "amino acid pool." Your body uses these amino acids the same way, regardless of whether they come from food or from your body.
3. Certain amino acids and glycerol from fat can be used to make glucose.
4. Products from glucose can be used in making both glycerol and some new amino acids (but not all amino acids).
5. The amino acids formed by the body, obtained from the breakdown of protein food, or obtained from the breakdown of body protein are used as needed to form new or additional body proteins.

Those who have more interest in what happens to food may have some

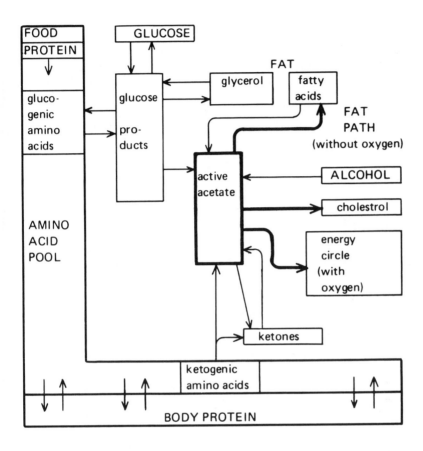

Fig. 33. Simplified concept of how protein, carbohydrate (glucose), fat, and alcohol are processed and interrelated in the metabolic system.

fun seeing how the whole processing line works together. You can consider the processing line like an ordinary road map. Let's call it the metabolic map. Watch the metabolic map, Figure 34, as you read through the discussion, and you can see all the different possibilities that can happen to your food. It will be just like many map game boards. Use it as if you were driving. Just follow the arrows from one location to the next on the metabolic map. You will see that some of these connections are two-way streets. Others are not.

Let's start on the metabolic map at glucose. Remember that all the carbohydrates in your food are glucose when they are finally prepared for

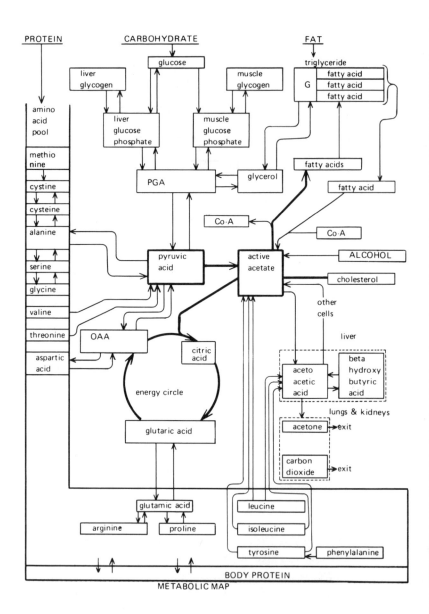

Fig. 34. The metabolic map.

use by cells. Starting at glucose you can follow the arrow to glucose phosphate, the first possible stop on the route. If you go to liver glucose phosphate you can take the turn and go to liver glycogen. This is a two-way street, and you can turn around and go back to liver glucose. The liver glucose phosphate can return to blood glucose. You could have taken the route to muscle glucose phosphate and from there to muscle glycogen. It is possible to return to muscle glucose phosphate. It is not possible to go all the way back to blood glucose because there is a one-way street from glucose to muscle glucose phosphate.

From either liver or muscle glucose phosphate you can go on down the route to PGA. This is a major intersection. From here you can follow the route to glycerol and then join the fatty acid stream of traffic to go to the fat depot. You could also come back out of the fat depot as glycerol and return to PGA using the two-way street. From PGA you can go on to pyruvic acid, and this is another major metabolic crossroad.

From pyruvic acid you can take the route to OAA. This is another busy metabolic intersection. When you get there note that this is the end of the two-way street. You can still turn around and trace your way all the way back to blood glucose or take any of the other routes to liver glycogen, muscle glycogen, glycerol or the fat depot.

Once you have arrived at OAA you can take the route to the fork in the road to meet with active acetate. Here two-carbon acetic acid is taken aboard and Co-A is released. You can take the route around the energy circle (citric-acid cycle). As you go around the circle, the two carbons from the acetic-acid passenger are ripped off one at a time, using oxygen and releasing energy. When you complete the energy circle, you are back where you started from, at OAA. You can go around and around the great energy circle, each time taking on a new acetic acid companion and ripping him apart. Or you could take any one of the other routes open from the OAA crossroad.

From OAA you can take on ammonia and become aspartic acid in the amino-acid pool. You are then in the heart of the great amino-acid exchange. This could lead to becoming part of a liver cell, part of an important hormone, or just a memory. The aspartic-acid route could lead to joining with other amino acids to form a purine base. This could be used to form DNA or RNA, the very life substance of the cells. The aspartic-acid route is a two-way street and you can follow the route back to OAA. From here you could take the route back to pyruvic acid.

From the pyruvic-acid junction there are several routes you could take. By adding an ammonia group to become alanine, you could go back to the amino-acid pool. This also is a two-way street. Or, you could follow the return route to blood glucose.

The other route you can follow is to the active-acetate corner. This is the hub of metabolic traffic flow. There's a lot of action here. But once you go the active-acetate route it is a no-return trip. You are locked into a limited portion of the metabolic route. From active acetate you can take the fat path forming new fatty acids and end up in the fat depot. That is temporary, though, and you can come back out and follow a different path to form active acetate again. Now you are back to the main acetate corner.

From the acetate corner you can take the route to cholesterol. This is the way a self-respecting glucose item from your food ends up as cholesterol. From here cholesterol can be recirculated in the bile over and over. Another route would be to form bile salts. The cholesterol could join the fatty particles in the bloodstream and go along the route to be deposited in the walls of arteries, causing atherosclerosis. This in turn can cause heart attacks, strokes, and other problems. The cholesterol could also be trapped with the food residue and discarded, taking it out of the metabolic traffic pattern, and out of the body. There is still another possible route from cholesterol. You could take the route to sex hormones, also formed from cholesterol—what a way to go! From sugar to sex.

From the acetate corner you could also take the ketone route. From here you could take the return trip (except through the liver and some other cells) back to the acetate corner. Or you could end up being eliminated in the urine or blown out in the breath as acetone. In either case, this is out of the metabolic system and out of the game. Still another choice from the acetate corner would be to make the big trip around the energy circle. This is it, though, you can only play once. From here you go to carbon dioxide, water, and energy.

Those, then, are the possible avenues you could take from glucose. It covers a lot of territory, from glucose to protein, fat, cholesterol, hormones, and bile salts. The list doesn't even end there. The acetate can also be used to detoxify toxic substances.

Now, let's look at the grand route for protein. If you enter the map from the protein access, you go to the amino-acid pool. If you take the route from glycine, the simplest amino acid, you can go back and forth to a number of other amino acids. One of these is alanine, or the route to pyruvic acid. Once at the pyruvic-acid junction you can take any of the routes described on the glucose itinerary. This means the route is open to fat, cholesterol, sex hormones, ketones, blood glucose, or energy.

Notice you can use alternate routes to go from one amino acid to another when a direct route is not available. You can go from aspartic acid to OAA, then on to pyruvic acid. From here you can go to alanine. This way you get from aspartic acid to alanine via pyruvic acid, but there is no direct route from aspartic acid to alanine.

You could take the amino-acid route via leucine, an essential amino acid. There is only a one-way route from here to the acetate corner or to the ketone tour. From the acetate corner you could do any of the tours out of acetate, but that is all. Since the body cannot make essential amino acids, you can't return. From the acetate corner, though, it is only a short trip to cholesterol and, finally, being lodged in a coronary artery, or even being a sex hormone. Since the essential-amino-acid route goes to the acetate corner, there is no way to go to either pyruvic acid or the OAA junction. This means the entire routes beyond these points are closed for essential amino acids. You can see, then, that essential amino acids tend to be ketogenic and the nonessential amino acids that have so much versatility tend to be glucogenic, that is, they can become glucose.

If you start out on the metabolic tour through the fat-access route, you can take the route to glycerol to PGA. From here it is possible to take any of the glucose tours. Remember, though, that only the glycerol from fat is an open route to glucose. The main fatty-acid route is direct to the acetate corner. From here the options are to return to fat via a different route, taking the cholesterol route or ketone route, or taking the energy circle (one trip to a customer). The fatty-acid route, then, doesn't include the many trips you can take through the glucose tour.

You can start on the metabolic map at the alcohol-access route. This is a direct channel to the acetate corner, and from here all the acetate routes to cholesterol and others are open.

Now you see all the possibilities of the metabolic processing system. It is entirely possible for glucose (from any carbohydrate source), protein, fat, or alcohol to become cholesterol, a ketone, a fat particle, or a sex hormone. As long as sufficient glucose is used, however, the normal body will not produce an excess amount of ketones.

When the metabolic route is overloaded, only a small amount of the traffic can go around the energy circle. The rest of the acetate units must take another route to ketones, to cholesterol, or to fat. To be broken down, ketones must also go around the energy circle. Normally, not many ketones are formed. It is little wonder, then, that when we overeat the system grinds out excess fat particles (triglycerides) and cholesterol, regardless of whether we are overeating from an excess intake of carbohydrates, fat, protein, or even alcohol.

This is an important concept, and it explains a lot of what goes on in the body with cholesterol and fatty particles. All that food must be processed some way. If only so much goes around the energy circle, the rest has to find another route. It is this "overflow of traffic" that is processed along the cholesterol route or along the fat path. There are two basic ways to slow down the formation of cholesterol and fatty particles. You can quit overloading the metabolic route with food. That will mean most of it can make it around the energy circle. Or you can increase the capacity of the energy circle. You do this by increasing the oxygen delivered by the circulation and by some stimulus like exercise. The exercise enables more food to be processed around the energy circle. This means there is less food that must take the fat path or the cholesterol route. You can see now why both diet control and exercise are important in preventing an excess formation of fatty particles and cholesterol.

14

DO YOU NEED CHOLINE AND LECITHIN?

There are a group of substances called *lipotropic factor* which are important in metabolic functions. The best-known of these are choline and lecithin. There are many people who regularly take lecithin tablets in the hope they will do great things for their health, including "dissolving fats and cholesterol." Let me say at once this trust in the value of lecithin tablets is not based on sound scientific facts. These substances are indeed necessary in the body, but the likelihood that your health will be greatly improved by taking these substances is small indeed. This is particularly true if you are eating a proper diet. It is sometimes claimed that the lecithin in egg yolks will neutralize the effects of the cholesterol in the yolk—this too is plain balderdash, a figment in yolk pigment.

Most of our information on what the lipotropic factor does comes from animal experiments, where a true choline deficiency or a deficiency in choline-producing substances was established. It is generally believed that such deficiencies can lead to fatty liver. And fatty liver occurs in conditions when a deficiency might be expected. The truth is that no one has demonstrated what degree of a deficiency or its duration must exist in man to produce these liver changes.

Globules of fat tend to be stored in the liver in excessive and abnormal amounts, sometimes causing liver damage and scarring or cirrhosis of the liver. Liver failure would be the final outcome. Fatty liver occurs on a very high-fat diet (a thought to keep in mind if you should contemplate some of those diets that depend on eating a lot of fat), in starvation, and in uncontrolled diabetes. In both starvation and diabetes the body lacks carbohydrates and the fat stores are mobilized and brought to the liver for processing to generate energy. For some reason the fat arrives faster than the liver can handle it, leading to the fatty-liver problem. Incidentally, you can also see this problem as a result of excessive prolonged use of alcohol. The diet in these circumstances is often deficient in lipotropic factor. Remember, too, that alcohol is metabolized through the acetate corner as a fat. Choline stimulates the liver to disassemble fatty acids. Without sufficient amounts the fat simply piles up in the liver.

Another serious complication of choline deficiency is hemorrhage in the kidneys. In rat experiments a deficient diet for five days resulted in severe high blood pressure from kidney damage four or five months later.

The problems induced by lipotropic deficiency are made worse by cholesterol, which among its other virtues is considered as an anti-lipotropic factor. Choline is readily absorbed from the intestine. It is not, however, absorbed from an ordinary diet in animals after the pancreas has been removed. Apparently the pancreatic enzymes are necessary to split off the choline from other food products before it can be absorbed. Choline can be manufactured by the body. All you need is sufficient amounts of the amino acids glycine and methionine. It is made up of carbon, hydrogen, nitrogen, and oxygen. By a simple chemical reaction they form choline. If your diet contains plenty of protein you should have enough choline.

How much choline do we need? Between 150 and 600 milligrams a day. Choline is present in large amounts in many common foods.

Choline per 100 Grams (3½ Ounces)

Lean meat	100 milligrams
Kidney	200 to 300
Brain	350 to 450
Liver	450 to 600
Fish	50 to 80
Whole eggs	35 to 700
Egg yolks	1400 to 1700
Cereals	50 to 100
Wheat germ	350 to 400

Vegetables are low in choline, fruit very low.

Choline does not exist in the body in a free state but rather is usually combined with a phospholipid, usually as lecithin. The lecithin in our body, however, doesn't get there by our swallowing lecithin tablets. These are simply torn down in the intestine before absorption is possible. The body puts together fatty acids (some of which may be polyunsaturated) with glycerol to form a triglyceride. One of the fatty-acid units is replaced by a phosphate—accomplished once more by using ATP. The phosphated fat then is hooked on to choline to form lecithin. You can think of lecithin as seen in Figure 35.

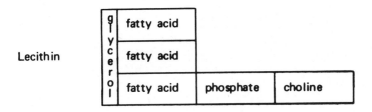

Fig. 35. Lecithin is fat, phosphate, and choline.

It should be kept in mind that to consume large amounts of lecithin is to consume fat and, while it usually comes from sources that contain polyunsaturated fat, it simply adds to the total fat intake. To decrease the cholesterol and fatty acids or triglycerides in the blood you will need to take other measures. It is true that the phospholipids increase the solubility of fats in the bloodstream, and lecithin is such a phospholipid combined with choline. However, the level of phospholipids depends on what the liver does with your overall food intake, rather than on the consumption of lecithin alone.

15

CONTROLLING YOUR
BLOOD SUGAR

A critical factor in how your metabolic functions work is the level of blood glucose. The blood level is important only because it is directly related to how much glucose gets in the cell. The action is inside the cell, not in the bloodstream. Regardless of what the level of blood glucose is, unless there is glucose inside the cell, it cannot be used for metabolic functions. Once glucose is in the cell it can be used for all the different things I've discussed. Among these is its ability to be processed to provide energy to run the body's complicated chemical system. Some of the nerve and brain cells, in particular, depend on glucose to provide energy for their complicated functions. If there is not enough glucose available inside the brain cells, normal brain function ceases. This can result in shock and even death.

In a person in good health, as the blood-glucose concentration rises more glucose will move across the cell membrane into the cell. As the blood-glucose level falls, less glucose will be available to cross the cell membrane and provide glucose for cell functions.

The amount of glucose in the blood is kept within fairly narrow limits to provide an optimal range of function in our bodies. The lower level can vary a great deal, even in healthy persons. Levels as low as 30 milligrams per cent (grams per 100 milliliters) have been reported in individuals who seemed to be functioning normally in all respects. This, however, is an unusually low level, and most people will begin to have difficulties when the blood-glucose level falls into the range of 40 or 50.

When the blood glucose rises too high, the excess amount is siphoned off by the kidney. In most healthy people, when the blood-glucose level exceeds 170 it begins to spill out into the urine. As long as the kidneys are able to eliminate the excess glucose rapidly, you should expect a range of 50 to 170, even in healthy people at different times in the day, depending on their habits.

In order to maintain the blood-glucose level, our body can use several different sources of glucose. The most obvious of these is to use carbohydrate in our diet to form blood glucose. In fact, most of the carbohydrates in our food are converted to glucose before they are absorbed through the intestinal wall into the bloodstream. Even drinking a concentrated solution of glucose water will only cause the blood-glucose level to rise a limited amount in healthy individuals. This is true despite the fact that the liquid solution can move immediately into the small intestine—particularly on an empty stomach, as in fasting tests of this nature. The glucose can be absorbed only so fast across the intestinal wall. This tends to limit the rate the blood-glucose level can rise. To cause a peak rise in the blood glucose, the rate of absorption of glucose through the intestinal wall would have to increase. Thyroid hormone speeds up absorption through the intestinal wall. It's not surprising, then, that individuals who have an overactive thyroid gland tend to have a sharp rise in the blood-sugar level after consuming concentrated amounts of glucose.

The degree of rise in the blood-glucose level can be controlled by limiting the amount of concentrated carbohydrates in the diet. Specifically, this means eliminating sweets and refined starches such as flour. Carbohydrates from sources that contain a lot of roughage, for example leafy vegetables, are emptied more slowly into the small intestine. The processing is so slow that the concentration of glucose in the liquid material that arrives in the small intestine never gets very high. With these relatively low concentrations of glucose in the food, the rate of absorption of glucose across the intestinal wall is slow. This helps to prevent the sharp peak rise in blood-glucose levels that occurs after taking sweet or syrupy foods.

Another source the body can call upon to raise the blood sugar is the liver glycogen. Remember that glycogen is just animal starch, and it's merely the way glucose units are packaged to be stored in the liver for future use. If the blood-glucose level falls, the liver simply breaks open packages of glycogen, processes it to glucose, and pours it out into the bloodstream. From here the glucose can be circulated to the innumerable cells in the body that can use the glucose for metabolic functions.

In the healthy individual who has been eating an adequate diet there should be about 100 grams (3½ ounces) of glycogen stored in the liver. This is enough under emergency situations to provide glucose for the body's needs for a period of two days. There is also a great deal of glycogen stored in the skeletal muscles. However, it is difficult, if not impossible, for this to be released back into the bloodstream and used by other organs, such as the brain, for its metabolic functions. It appears, for the most part, to be trapped within the muscle fibers. It can be converted to glucose phosphate within the muscles and then used for the metabolic actions in the muscle fibers. This store of glycogen in the muscles is immediately available for sudden physical exertion.

As you've seen from the discussion of how the body processes your food, there is still another way the body can provide glucose for its needs. A number of the amino acids from the protein in the food can be stripped of their ammonia group and converted to glucose through the metabolic processing line. This formation of new glucose from other substances is called gluconeogenesis (birth of new glucose). If a person doesn't have sufficient liver glycogen or carbohydrate in the diet, mixed protein intake can be used to provide glucose. The body isn't too discriminating either. It can take these proteins from the diet or from the body, including the muscle cells. Dietary protein then, and even the protein stores in the body, can be used in an emergency situation to provide blood glucose. This can then be used as energy for the essential body functions necessary to maintain life. You should keep this point in mind when you think about diets that are extremely low or entirely lacking in carbohydrates.

As you know from studying the metabolic map and from discussions of the metabolic role of amino acids, not all of them can be converted to glucose. A number of the essential amino acids are ketogenic, which means they can become ketone bodies, but they can't be used to form glucose. Nevertheless, these amino acids can be used to provide energy once they have been converted to active acetate to be processed around the energy circle; they thereby decrease the need for the body to use glucose for energy. Even those amino acids that are ketogenic can be thought of as "glucose sparing" if they are used as a source of energy. This clearly means that on a no-carbohydrate diet even essential amino acids can be destroyed to provide the body's needed energy. This, of course, is a very wasteful and inefficient way of providing energy.

Your body can also use glycerol to form glucose. Remember, the glycerol can be split off from fat and enter the glucose metabolic route to become blood glucose. Or it can take the other turn and go all the way to OAA to be used to provide a means to operate the energy circle. The glycerol in 100 grams of fat provides 12 grams of glucose.

It is important to realize that neither fatty acids nor alcohol can be used to increase the blood-glucose level. Both go through the metabolic route to the active-acetate corner in the traffic pattern. From this corner there is no way to take the route to pyruvic acid, or in any other way to gain access to the remainder of the glucose processing line. The only way fatty acids or alcohol can help in maintaining the blood-glucose level is that they can be used for energy, and so decrease the necessity for the cells to use glucose for energy. There must be sufficient OAA available to take the acetate units around the energy circle to provide energy. Remember that the brain and some other cells require glucose to operate their metabolic system and carry out their normal functions.

Obviously if the body is to maintain the glucose level within a narrow range, it needs not only a source of glucose but also a way of eliminating excess amounts. There are several ways in which the blood-glucose level can be lowered. First on this list, of course, is the formation of glycogen. A limited amount of glucose can be stored in the liver and muscles in this form for future use.

A second mechanism of lowering the blood-glucose level is through the expenditure of energy, which involves the use of oxygen to operate the energy circle. A good example would be physical activity. In running, the muscles must have energy for mechanical work. Increased amounts of oxygen are delivered by the circulation to the working muscles using the oxygen. Glucose is processed around the energy circle to yield energy for the mechanical action. In this way, glucose is rapidly used up. After prolonged heavy exertion, the blood-glucose level tends to fall, unless additional glucose is poured into the system. It's been demonstrated that a dog's work capacity can be increased by giving him small amounts of glucose during long periods of heavy physical exertion, as during treadmill exercise. The same applies to man. A spoonful of sugar literally makes the work go on.

A third way to lower the blood-glucose level is to convert the glucose to fat. This is accomplished by converting the glucose to active acetate. From there the fat path is used to form fatty acids. These are combined with glycerol and the fatty particle is deposited.

A fourth way of decreasing the blood-glucose level is simply to filter the glucose out through the kidneys. Normally this system is used when the glucose level gets fairly high, usually around 170 or more. Under these circumstances the blood-glucose level is rising faster than the body can process it. As a result, the glucose is lost.

There are some less important ways of losing glucose. Remember, glucose can become active acetate and then cholesterol. You could lose glucose through the elimination of cholesterol with the food residue. A certain amount of cholesterol is always eliminated from the body this way. In rare cases, the kidneys will have a defect and spill glucose into the urine, even when the blood-glucose level is normal.

The job of maintaining the balance between glucose taken out and glucose poured into the blood is the duty of the liver. Just as a thermostat regulates heat, the liver may be thought of as the "glucostat" to regulate the level of the blood glucose. It increases blood glucose when it's needed, primarily through the use of liver glycogen and gluconeogenesis. It lowers the blood-glucose level when it gets too high by making glycogen and forming fatty acids.

A number of factors influence the metabolic scheme to control the blood-glucose level. The hormone insulin is a major one. Insulin is formed by tiny specialized endocrine-gland tissue located in small islands within the pancreas. Insulin is a protein, and it is released into the bloodstream. From here it is carried throughout the body by the circulation. Its most important function is to assist in transferring the glucose into the cell. Without sufficient insulin available at the cell, it will be difficult to move glucose into the cell. This in turn means glucose won't be available for normal cell function, at least in its usual quantities. Since the movement of glucose into the cell depends on the blood-glucose level, our body responds to a lack of insulin by raising the level of blood glucose. This helps to increase the amount of glucose that can be moved into the cells for cell functions.

The effect of insulin is to lower the blood-glucose level. By helping to get the glucose into the cells, it obviously increases the use of glucose, lowering the level in the blood. Insulin also helps to lower the blood glucose by stimulating the formation of glycogen. If not much insulin is available, it will be difficult to form glycogen in the liver. Finally, insulin increases the conversion of glucose to fatty acids by actively promoting fatty-acid formation. All three of these actions—increasing the use of glucose by the cells, increasing the formation of glycogen, and increasing the conversion of glucose to fatty acids—tend to lower blood glucose. The role of insulin in facilitating the conversion of active acetate to fatty acids is the basis for many comments about the role of insulin in obesity.

Insulin also acts to prevent a rise in blood glucose. It does this by inhibiting the conversion of amino acids to glucose. In this way its actions spare body protein by preventing the use of amino acids to form blood glucose. Insulin may also help to prevent the conversion of glycogen to glucose, conserving these stores of emergency energy for other purposes.

There is evidence that low insulin levels tend to promote the mobilization of fat. This is of interest to people who are interested in having their fat mobilized as part of a weight-reducing program. It should be pointed out, however, that with the mobilization of body fat there is sharp increase in blood-fat levels. If this is maintained over long periods of time, it may contribute to formation of cholesterol-containing fatty particles within the walls of the arteries and the development of atherosclerosis. It is the action of insulin in preventing the mobilization of fat that can be considered as preventing atherosclerosis.

The combination of the actions of insulin to prevent the use of amino acids to form glucose and to facilitate the use of glucose rather than other substances for energy means insulin is important in promoting body-tissue growth. In short, it's important in developing and maintaining muscle mass and the strength that accompanies this.

Many complex factors influence how much insulin is released into our bodies. Whenever the blood-glucose level rises, insulin will be poured out into the bloodstream. Sometimes after one eats carbohydrate, the insulin level in the bloodstream may increase seven to ten times within an hour. After a few hours, the level returns to normal. In case an individual has no food for twenty-four to forty-eight hours the insulin level begins to fall, sometimes to undetectable levels. From what I've already told you about the role of insulin in mobilizing fat, it should be clear that at these very low blood levels of insulin fat mobilization would be more likely. This makes sense because it would then be necessary for the body to use fats for energy. Before the fat can be used for energy, it has to be mobilized out of the fat cells and carried to the tissues for metabolic processing.

Insulin does not have uncontested influence over the blood-glucose level. Our body has a group of checks and balances. The pituitary gland just below the brain pours out a hormone which essentially is an anti-insulin hormone. You can think of the pituitary hormone as neutralizing insulin. The two hormones have opposite actions. They help regulate the actions in the liver to maintain an optimal range of blood glucose.

Whenever you eat anything which causes the blood-glucose level to rise, there will be a sharp decrease in the amount of pituitary hormone released. Eating increases insulin release. If the blood-glucose level falls too much, there will be an outpouring of pituitary hormone to raise the blood-glucose level. In contrast, as the blood-glucose level falls, insulin formation is sharply curtailed. These two hormones act together to stabilize the blood-glucose levels. Immediately after eating, insulin is released into the bloodstream to lower the blood-glucose level, and production of the pituitary hormone is slowed. This achieves the goal of lowering the blood-glucose level. Later, as the level begins to plummet, insulin formation is curtailed, and pituitary hormone production is increased. The main action of the pituitary hormone is to increase the conversion of amino acids to glucose. It stimulates the release of fatty acids from fat depots so these can be used instead of glucose, thus sparing the blood glucose for essential needs.

Between these two extremes of action, there is an optimal range when both insulin and pituitary hormones are present in moderate amounts. At this level they act together to stimulate growth, tissue formation, and production of protein substances. Both insulin and pituitary hormone are necessary for normal growth-promoting activity. It has been demonstrated in animals that you can remove both the pituitary and the pancreas, eliminating both pituitary hormone and insulin. Surprisingly enough the blood-glucose levels will stay in fairly normal ranges, but the animal loses its safety mechanism and responds more drastically to factors that would normally increase or lower blood-glucose levels. His body's response becomes jerky, lacking smooth coordination.

It's worth noting here that a factor in the pituitary hormones has the capacity to mobilize fatty acids. This has caused a great deal of interest in using various hormones to assist in weight-reducing programs. While these systems operate normally within sets of checks and balances within the body, their applicability in weight-reduction programs is open to serious question. It may be, however, that as blood-glucose levels fall because of diet restriction, the increased pituitary hormone release and decreased insulin release act together to help mobilize fatty acids for energy. This, in turn, can lead to a significant rise in blood-fat levels, a condition that some medical specialists consider detrimental to health, at least on a relatively long-term basis.

The blood-glucose level is also affected by hormones from the adrenal cortex, the outer shell of the little gland that rests above each kidney. These powerful hormones of the cortisone group are used in many medical problems. The adrenal cortex hormones should be considered as basically anti-insulin hormones. They act by stimulating the liver to convert amino acids to glucose, raising the blood-glucose level. They also seem to slow down or inhibit the use of glucose in the cells, which tends to cause a rise in blood-glucose levels. It's not too surprising, then, that individuals who have poorly functioning adrenal glands, with decreased hormone formation, as seen in Addison's disease, tend to have low blood-glucose levels. These people are particularly sensitive to insulin.

Adrenaline, our fight-or-flight hormone, is formed in the center of the adrenal gland. It causes the body to break down glycogen or specially packaged glucose stores to glucose to be utilized for energy. This is a very rapid process, and mobilizing these stores for energy gives rise to the concept that adrenaline prepares our body for fight or flight. It's important to realize that when the blood glucose falls, the adrenal gland is stimulated to pour out adrenaline. This is a major factor in causing a number of the symptoms experienced by people with genuine low blood glucose.

Still another hormone, glucagon, is thought to increase the blood-glucose level, probably by breaking down glycogen into glucose. Glucagon is formed in the same islets of tissues that form insulin. The extent of its role in our body, though, has not been fully defined. We know it's present and may be a factor in some instances, but how often it's important in regulating blood glucose in man and diseases of man is not fully appreciated at this time.

You can think of the effects of the various hormones that regulate the blood glucose level as a simple balance-scale system (see Figure 36).

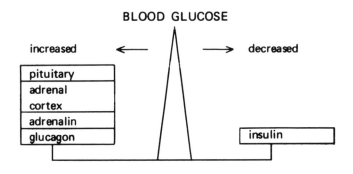

Fig. 36. The blood glucose depends upon the balance of several hormones.

On one side of the balance scales are pituitary hormones, adrenal cortical hormones, and adrenaline, all of which tip the scale toward an increase in the blood-glucose level. These are all, in a sense, anti-insulin hormones. On the other side of the balance scale is insulin, which tends to tip the balance in the direction of decreased blood glucose.

With the body's ability to use amino acids to form glucose, the use of glycerol to form glucose, and the use of fatty acids for energy instead of glucose, there are many ways in which the glucose level can be maintained. Similarly, the body's ability to convert glucose to fat or cholesterol, or tear it down for energy, or even to form glycogen provides numerous ways in which the blood-glucose level can be lowered. The body has many alternatives in maintaining the blood glucose at a level suitable for optimal metabolic functions of the cells.

16

WHY DIABETICS ARE TIRED

Diabetes is a metabolic disturbance that has afflicted man since well before the time of Christ. It was described in the first century A.D. in medical writings as a "melting down of the flesh and limbs to urine." Briefly, diabetes is a disease associated with a high blood-glucose level and an inability of the body to use glucose. This isn't the total picture, though. A lot more happens to a person with true diabetes than just failure to utilize glucose properly. Furthermore, many problems besides diabetes can cause abnormal elevations of blood glucose. Nevertheless, one of the best indicators of the presence of diabetes is a persistent, abnormal elevation of the blood glucose.

By analogy, diabetes can be thought of as an insulin deficiency. In fact, insulin remains the most useful form of therapy in treating diabetics. Diabetes is caused by the failure of insulin to facilitate the movement of glucose into the cell. Because of this the blood-glucose level is increased to help glucose across the cell membrane into the cell for metabolic action. The elevated blood-glucose level, then, is an indicator that something is wrong in the normal insulin mechanism needed to enable the body adequately to use glucose.

A common way of evaluating the presence or absence of diabetes is by performing a glucose-tolerance test; this test measures how the body handles glucose. The stomach must be empty for the examination. The patient drinks 100 grams of glucose dissolved in water. As you know from the discussions on emptying of the stomach, this means that the glucose rapidly enters the small intestine. Here it is absorbed at a fairly constant rate. The amount of glucose in the blood is determined before the patient drinks the glucose water and at timed intervals thereafter.

The blood-glucose level in the fasting state can vary a great deal. It can be moderately elevated, just from such factors as stress before a medical examination. Even so, it's decidedly unusual for the fasting level to be higher than 125 grams per 100 milliliters. Values higher than this are usually associated with abnormal metabolic processing of glucose. In individuals with moderate or mild diabetes the fasting blood-glucose level may be entirely normal. You can tell there's a problem only by the body's response after the glucose is ingested.

Glucose water, just like any other syrupy drink that accumulates in the intestine, is absorbed at a fairly uniform rate into the bloodstream. Although water is rapidly absorbed from the small intestine, this is not true of glucose. Its maximum absorption rate maintains a steady, continuous addition of glucose to the bloodstream. This tends to prevent too sharp a rise in the blood-glucose level from eating. In healthy individuals the blood-glucose level usually doesn't rise much over 170. This occurs often enough, however. This is near the level that glucose is spilled out in the urine. It's not uncommon to see a small amount of sugar in the urine after drinking or eating large amounts of glucose.

In the diabetic, because the glucose is not being utilized, the blood-glucose level may rise much higher than 170. In healthy people the glucose in the blood is rapidly dispatched either into the cells for the energy process or converted to glycogen and stored or otherwise processed by the metabolic machinery. As a result, within two hours after the glucose water has been ingested the blood-glucose level will be down to 120 or even lower. Not infrequently it's back to the fasting level. Because the diabetic can't use the glucose it continues to circulate about in the bloodstream, and the high blood-glucose level will persist for hours.

The characteristic response of a moderately severe diabetic to drinking glucose water is a high fasting blood glucose, an abnormally high rise after drinking the glucose, and a persistently high level over two hours. Diabetics who do not have quite such a severe problem may have a normal fasting blood-glucose level, with an abnormally high rise that persists beyond two hours after ingesting glucose.

Because so many mild or moderate diabetics have a normal fasting blood glucose a fasting test is not a reliable screening test for diabetes. You may have had blood tests done at the time of your medical examination to check for diabetes. If all the blood samples were drawn in the fasting state it's unlikely that such a testing procedure will discover mild diabetes even if you have it. A better screening test is to obtain a blood sample two hours after eating or after drinking glucose water. Far more diabetic problems will be detected by this test than from a simple fasting blood sample. Of course, if either test is suspicious most specialists prefer to perform a complete glucose-tolerance test. They may want other tests as well to be certain that the problem really is diabetes.

Our bodies are remarkable in their ability to adapt to what we do. A common cause for an elevated blood-glucose level that resembles diabetes in testing is a calorie-restricted diet. With so many people on diets to reduce their weight, this is a frequent problem in the doctor's office. If your body is not receiving a reasonable amount of carbohydrate regularly, it doesn't pour out as much insulin as it normally would. It literally loses its ability to manufacture insulin. The loss is only temporary and is a matter of function. It's closely akin to the old biological principle, "If you don't use it, you lose it." If you don't need to have a lot of insulin poured out into the bloodstream, it's not going to be manufactured. As soon as you start consuming a reasonable amount of carbohydrates, causing a significant rise in the blood-glucose level, the body will get used to manufacturing insulin and releasing it when your system needs it. The situation is actually a bit more complicated than that and involves a number of enzyme systems, but you can use this as a working explanation of how this phenomenon occurs.

For years I examined many healthy U.S. Air Force pilots. They came to the Aerospace Medical Center for such things as evaluation for the astronaut program. Often they had been on a diet for several days to get rid of some excess pounds before their physical exam. The results were predictable. Their metabolic mechanisms designed to handle carbohydrate loads had become relatively dormant. Some of them demonstrated an abnormal response to glucose water, similar to that seen in a diabetic. These same men were then placed on a high-carbohydrate diet. After only three days their mechanisms to process glucose were activated and they would have a normal glucose test just like anyone else.

The moral of the story is simple. If you're going to have a medical evaluation, unless you're already a diabetic or there are other problems involved, you ought to prepare yourself by eating a good, normal, adequate diet for at least three days before the examination. Of course most individuals have to be fasting when they report to the laboratory. That won't keep you from eating a good, normal, balanced diet with adequate amounts of carbohydrate for at least three days before the overnight fast for the examination.

Another cause for high blood-glucose levels in testing is the presence of an overactive pituitary gland. If excess amounts of pituitary hormone are being formed, they can literally neutralize the effects of insulin and cause a diabetic response. Such a problem can be seen in the rare individual who has a hormone-secreting pituitary tumor.

The uncontrolled diabetic commonly has "sugar in the urine." The sweet urine is caused by the spilling over of the excess glucose through the kidneys into the urine. If the kidneys are normal the blood-glucose level was over 160 or 170 at some point in time. Obviously the higher and the more persistently high the blood-glucose levels are, the more glucose will be lost in the urine. If a person has emptied his bladder completely and then remains in the fasting state and continues to show glucose in the urine, he usually has diabetes. For this reason, the first morning urine specimen in a fasting person that contains sugar may well be indicative of diabetes. But sugar in the urine alone should not be used as a diagnosis for diabetes. Rather, a more complete examination, including blood tests, is necessary to establish this. Even so, tests for the amounts of sugar in the urine are helpful in guiding patients in the home management of their diabetes. It's important again to emphasize that nondiabetic people can have sugar in the urine. All that needs to happen is for them to absorb a large load of glucose into the bloodstream. If the blood-glucose level is too high, even momentarily, the kidney acts as an overflow valve and it spills out in the urine.

In an uncontrolled diabetic all that glucose concentrated in the urine creates a problem. In fact, the kidneys have limited ability to concentrate glucose and must dilute it with a considerable amount of water. The diluted "sugar water" results in the formation of large amounts of urine. Doctors like to call this polyuria. Anyone who has this symptom is well aware of it because he will be making frequent trips to the bathroom. The person who is nervous or has inflammation of the bladder, prostate trouble, or similar problems runs to the bathroom frequently to eliminate small amounts of urine. The diabetic eliminates a lot of urine each trip. Not only that, the process will continue at night.

Anyone who is losing a lot of water in his urine will have to replace it to preserve the balance of water in the body. This results in a horrendous thirst in the diabetic, so he's always complaining of being thirsty and drinking lots of water or other fluids. Eliminating all that water, plus the high blood-glucose level, drains water out of the cells. As a result, it's common for the uncontrolled diabetic to have a water deficit within his cells. This can contribute to additional disturbances in the salt, mineral, and water balance of the body.

In addition to the problems of passing a lot of urine and extreme thirst, the diabetic often experiences extreme fatigue. In fact, fatigue is sometimes the first symptom to bring the diabetic to the doctor's office. Having read about our energy system, you can easily understand this. Energy to run the body depends on stripping the food elements of their energy within the cell itself. If the glucose can't get into the cell to be processed, glucose is no longer available to provide energy to run the body. Quite naturally, fatigue occurs. Even the building process from amino acids, from which you might expect to get some help, is diminished because without sufficient insulin many of the amino acids are used to form more glucose. This glucose can't be used by the body any better than glucose taken from glycogen or your food sources.

This means the untreated severe diabetic will have to depend largely on fat and ketogenic amino acids for energy. It's not surprising, then, that uncontrolled, moderately severe diabetes is associated with mobilizing any fat stores the body has. It's not uncommon for a diabetic to have been reasonably overweight originally. As the diabetes becomes more severe, the excess fat deposits are mobilized and used for energy. Remember, insulin inhibits the mobilization of fat and is used in the manufacture of fatty acids. When not enough insulin is available the fat is mobilized. In addition, the ability to form fatty acids from active acetate derived from either glucose or amino acids is defective.

Diabetes is one of those curious circumstances in which more fat is mobilized than the liver can process. It causes the body to behave very much as if you were on a high-fat diet; and little wonder, since fat has become the principal source of energy. It's particularly important that the diabetic have an adequate amount of lipotropic factor in the diet. That means choline or substances such as amino acids, methionine, and glycine to provide choline. The uncontrolled diabetic tends to accumulate abnormal, excessive amounts of fat in the liver. This can cause liver damage, scarring, and cirrhosis. Liver damage is a frequent complication of diabetes, particularly if the diabetes is not adequately controlled.

The blood-fat levels, and incidentally the cholesterol levels, are often abnormally elevated in the diabetic. This is caused partly by the mobilization of fat for energy and can lead to an increased formation of cholesterol within the walls of the arteries throughout the body. Diabetics are particularly prone to atherosclerosis with the complicating problems of heart attacks, strokes, and poor circulation to the feet. The latter leads to diabetic gangrene. The overall high fat level and high sugar levels damage the arteries and the kidneys. Abnormal kidney function is another frequent complication of uncontrolled diabetes.

In the moderately severe diabetic, inadequately treated, the body must depend on using fat and those amino acids that go the route of fat metabolism for energy. This leads to the production of large amounts of ketones, the acetoacetic-acid group that comes from active acetate. These can accumulate in very large amounts. They are highly acid and tend to upset the body's salt, mineral, and water balance as they are eliminated.

Acetone may be formed in large amounts and eliminated through the lungs. This accounts for the acetone breath of the uncontrolled diabetic. When ketones are produced more rapidly than they can be processed through the energy circle, their level builds up, sometimes producing a serious disturbance in the chemical balance of the body, a condition called acidosis. This can cause diabetic coma, shock, and death. Diabetic coma is a severe medical emergency requiring immediate treatment.

Now you can begin to appreciate why the diabetic has severe weight loss. If the disease progresses without control, weight loss occurs even though the appetite may be quite good. In severe states there may be as much as 500 grams of glucose, or 2000 calories a day, lost in the urine. All this glucose doesn't have to come from carbohydrates from the diet either. A good part of the protein that's eaten can also be converted to glucose and be eliminated in the urine. Thus, severe, uncontrolled diabetes puts a severe strain on the protein sources from both the food and the body and makes it impossible to use carbohydrates. With all this loss of calories through the urine it's little wonder the severe diabetic loses weight. The weight loss can involve a mobilization and use of fat deposits, but it also can go to the point of causing loss of protein stores in the muscles.

Now you can form a picture of the advanced diabetic and have a pretty good idea of how diabetes works on your metabolic map. Such an individual frequently eliminates large amounts of urine. He is thirsty, fatigued, eats a lot and is still thin or even loses weight. If the condition is allowed to progress, you can smell the acetone on his breath—it smells as if he has been drinking. As the ketones build up, disorientation, acidosis, and coma can follow.

The most successful form of treatment of severe diabetics is the use of insulin. By giving the appropriate amount of insulin, the utilization of glucose is increased and all those symptoms I just mentioned begin to be reversed. Insulin enables the diabetic to use glucose for energy whether it comes from carbohydrates or from certain amino acids. In this sense it promotes the development of body protein, including protein for all the vital hormones and enzyme systems needed for the body's normal function. In general, the total function of the body's biological system is markedly improved. The blood-glucose levels decrease with adequate control, and loss of energy through the urine is slowed and eventually stopped.

There is considerable debate, even among experts, as to how well the blood-glucose level needs to be controlled. Many individuals like to keep the level reasonably low. Others feel that this is a bit ritualistic. Almost all experts would agree, however, that it's wise to keep the blood-glucose level low enough that large amounts of energy in the form of glucose are not lost in the urine.

What about the diet for a diabetic? You can obtain many different answers to this question, but in truth there is no standard diabetic diet. Many obese individuals with moderately elevated blood glucose have normal glucose test results after they lose their excess body fat. In general, an obese person with high blood-glucose levels can be helped with a good sensible diet directed toward eliminating obesity. After adequate weight reduction many of these individuals only need an adequate diet and weight-control program.

Beyond weight control, the diet needs to be adapted for the individual. We can make certain generalizations. It is true, within limits, that consuming concentrated sweets and starches will cause a more rapid rise in the blood-glucose level than other foods. The amounts of these should be limited to help the diabetic avoid peak increases in blood glucose that might not be adequately covered by the insulin he may be taking. Expressed another way, a large portion of the carbohydrates in the diet should come from bulk carbohydrates, specifically those in vegetables and whole cereals.

There is no valid reason for a diabetic not to have carbohydrates in the diet. Avoiding them will not help the diabetic condition. After all, the body can manufacture its own glucose even from its own protein. In case you've heard that eating a lot of carbohydrates will cause diabetes, that's not true—at least if you eliminate the individuals who are simply overweight with high glucose levels. In many populations where a large portion of the calorie intake is from starch there is no higher incidence of diabetes than there is in populations where this is not the case.

The diet of a diabetic should certainly contain adequate amounts of protein. Even eating large amounts of protein, however, won't enable the body to produce protein for body development and protein production in uncontrolled diabetes.

In the past it has been advocated that diabetics include a lot of fat in their diet while cutting down on their carbohydrates. There doesn't seem to be any valid reason for this, particularly if the disease can be controlled adequately with proper insulin treatment. In fact, because diabetics are prone to develop atherosclerosis and mobilize fat from the body it's probably not a very good idea. It may be necessary to have an appreciable amount of fat in the diet just to survive if the individual has moderately severe diabetes and is not going to be treated medically. In this situation fat is the major energy source. But no one recommends this approach in the treatment of diabetes; that is, eating fat alone without carbohydrates and not using insulin.

The one thing that should be stressed for the diabetic who must be on a diet and requires insulin is that he follow his diet carefully and exactly. The amount of insulin the diabetic needs is dependent in large measure on what he eats. In the nondiabetic person the amount of insulin needed is automatically adjusted to what he eats. The severe diabetic doesn't have this ability. The artificial means of providing insulin by needle requires that the food and the insulin input be synchronized. If this is not done, insulin may be provided to the bloodstream at a time the blood-glucose level is already normal. This can cause an abnormally low glucose level. Then the insulin won't be available when the glucose level goes up with subsequent eating. For this reason, dietary habits, which include not only the amount but timing of eating, and the insulin administration should be a fairly regular routine.

This comment about the diet and insulin also applies to the other life habits. Diabetics need to regulate their habits so there will not be unusual metabolic stresses that the body can't cope with. A good illustration here is exercise. Marked physical activity, even in the diabetic, tends to increase the use of glucose in the cells as long as this mechanism is intact at all. As a result, athletic competition, physical exercise, or just hard labor may increase the utilization of blood glucose. Unless the insulin dosage is decreased or the carbohydrate intake is increased, the blood-glucose level may fall too low. In general, then, the diabetic should have a good, nutritious diet, adequate in protein, vitamins, minerals, and all essential nutrients. It should contain the proper number of calories for that individual to maintain optimal nutrition. And it should be standardized in relationship to the rest of the treatment program.

17

LOW BLOOD SUGAR
AND YOUR ENERGY

Other than obesity, probably no metabolic problem has received more popular attention than "low blood sugar," properly called hypoglycemia. Hypoglycemia has become a popular diagnosis. In many respects it is a catchall wastebasket for a variety of symptoms that can be caused by hypoglycemia but are also caused by many other problems.

Even the definition of hypoglycemia is confusing. You'd think it would mean low blood glucose, but the arguments begin as soon as you try to define how low the glucose level must be for the label. The real crux of the problem is that the level of glucose in the blood is relatively unimportant. What counts is the level of glucose in the cells, where it can be utilized for metabolic function. It has been reported that healthy individuals have even been able to tolerate blood-glucose levels as low as 30 for short periods of time without any evidence of difficulties.

Most scientific papers state that if the level in a healthy person is below 50 grams per 100 milliliters, the person will probably show symptoms of hypoglycemia. I must say from personal experience, however, that endurance athletes trained for the Olympics commonly have levels lower than 50, although they are in optimal health with abundant energy and exhibit no symptoms of hypoglycemia. Adelle Davis wrote that the fasting "blood sugar" is 90 to 95, that at levels of 70 "hunger is experienced, and lassitude gradually becomes fatigue." Because doctors see patients and have clinical experience, they know that normal healthy people with plenty of energy commonly have levels of 70. Such a fixation on numbers has little or no relation to biological reality. Such nonsense, available to the public, has a lot to do with the general mistaken ideas about "low blood sugar."

Under special circumstances the blood-glucose levels can be abnormally high and still be associated with a low cell-glucose level, causing all the symptoms of low blood glucose. A severe diabetic, for example, may require a blood-glucose level of over 150 to facilitate the movement of glucose into the cell. If the blood-glucose level fell below 150 in such a diabetic, there would be a diminished supply of glucose in the cell, producing symptoms of low blood glucose. At best, then, the blood-glucose level is only a guide to what might be going on.

Because of the widespread confusion about low blood glucose the *Journal of the American Medical Association* published an official statement:

> Recent publicity in the popular press has led the public to believe that the occurrence of hypoglycemia is widespread in this country and that many of the symptoms that affect the American population are not recognized as being caused by this condition. These claims are not supported by medical evidence. Because of the possible misunderstanding about the matter, three organizations of physicians and scientists (the American Diabetes Association, the Endocrine Society, and the American Medical Association) have issued the following statement for the public concerning the diagnosis and treatment of hypoglycemia:

>> Hypoglycemia means a low level of blood glucose. When it occurs, it is often attended by symptoms of sweating, shakiness, trembling, anxiety, fast heart action, headache, hunger sensations, brief feelings of weakness, and occasionally, seizures and coma. However, the majority of people with these kinds of symptoms do not have hypoglycemia; a great many patients with anxiety reactions present with similar symptoms. Furthermore, there is no good evidence that hypoglycemia causes depression, chronic fatigue, allergies, nervous breakdowns, alcoholism, juvenile delinquency, childhood behavior problems, drug addiction or inadequate sexual performance. . . .

This statement from the American Medical Association is at least symptomatic of the level of confusion that has been introduced about low blood glucose. As we discuss the metabolic derangements associated with low blood glucose, you can see the basis for some of these statements.

There are several ways that symptoms of low blood glucose can be produced. One of these is the direct effect of inadequate amounts of glucose in the cells of the brain. The brain is particularly dependent upon glucose for its functions. When it doesn't have enough, mental confusion occurs. This can even be associated with hallucinations, aimless excessive activity, convulsions, and coma. Giving large amounts of insulin to induce insulin shock or low blood glucose was once a common treatment in a number of psychiatric hospitals. Very low blood-glucose levels can cause poor function of localized areas of the brain causing temporary paralysis of one or more limbs and symptoms closely resembling a stroke. If the low blood-glucose level is sufficiently prolonged, and of sufficient severity, it can even cause permanent damage to the brain cortex.

Low blood glucose also causes symptoms by stimulating the body to pour out adrenaline. Whenever our blood-glucose level falls too low, a signal is relayed to the adrenal gland to pour out the adrenaline. Remember, adrenaline causes our animal starch or glycogen to be unpackaged to dump glucose into the blood system. The release of adrenaline is our body's reaction to protect us against a severely low blood-glucose level. The problem is that a large amount of adrenaline causes a lot of other changes besides increasing the blood glucose. It will significantly affect the heart, causing it to beat rapidly, sometimes with heart pounding. There is no question about it, excessive amounts of adrenaline will create a feeling of anxiety and cause a person to become pale and sweaty. The blood pressure also rises. It is this pale, sweaty, anxious state with rapidly beating heart that alerts many people to the presence of low blood glucose.

I hasten to add there are many other conditions that will cause adrenaline to be released. One is simple fright. After all, it's the hormone to prepare us for fight or flight. Anxiety of any type, including chronic recurring anxiety, can cause an outpouring of adrenaline and produce these symptoms. Basically what the American Medical Association's statement is saying is that there are a lot more individuals with anxiety than there are those whose symptoms are really caused by low blood sugar.

I want to emphasize that a low blood-glucose level is merely a symptomatic finding. It is not a diagnosis. Also, the symptoms associated with the adrenaline response are just that, symptoms of an adrenaline response. It remains for the doctor to find out what's causing it—anxiety, a real case of low blood glucose (and, if so, what's causing that), or some other factor.

In addition to these symptoms, actual low blood glucose will commonly induce hunger. People who have problems with low blood glucose soon learn that their symptoms, including those induced by the pouring out of adrenaline, and their hunger can be relieved by eating something sweet. As a result they often continually eat sweet foods. The little center in the brain, often referred to as the appestat, that affects our appetite has a lot to do with our sensation of hunger. There is considerable evidence that it is sensitive to the blood-glucose level. It is activated when the blood-glucose level falls too low and causes us to have the sensation of hunger. It is satisfied and turns off our hunger sensation when the blood-glucose level rises sufficiently. It's not surprising, then, that low blood glucose is often associated with hunger sensations.

Hypoglycemia also stimulates the stomach, through reflex mechanisms, to pour out acid pepsin juice. In persons with sensitive mechanisms this can cause nausea and symptoms of acid stomach. These may be more noticeable than hunger sensations.

Many individuals who have low-blood-glucose problems also have an obesity problem. The continual eating to try to shore up the blood-glucose level results in a high calorie intake. I'm often reminded of a patient I first saw in medical school who had low blood glucose because of a tumor in the pancreas that was producing excessive amounts of insulin. He ate large quantities of food and was very obese. After his tumor had been removed, curing him of his problem, he lost his excess weight and became an ordinary, lean, vigorous individual. Most cases of obesity are not the result of low blood glucose or an overproduction of insulin. More often obesity is directly caused simply by eating too much in relation to the individual's level of physical activity and other metabolic functions. The overeating is related to habits and environmental and emotional factors.

Because insulin may induce low blood glucose and is essential in the formation of fatty acids, some believe insulin contributes to obesity. No doubt its presence is necessary since clearly the severe diabetic who has a gross deficiency in insulin function tends to lose weight. To extend this idea to some mystical overproduction of insulin as the major cause of obesity is not based on sound studies.

The victim of low blood glucose often complains of fatigue just as the diabetic does and, interestingly enough, for the same reason. For the body to use glucose for energy the glucose has to get into the cell. Obviously, if the blood-glucose level is too low, there won't be enough glucose in the cell. Similarly, in a severe diabetic, not adequately treated, there won't be an adequate insulin mechanism to transfer glucose into the cell, so he won't have glucose available for energy either. Fatigue is a prominent symptom of both conditions. On the surface it seems paradoxical that one patient with a high blood-glucose level will be fatigued, and at the other end of the spectrum the patient with very low blood glucose will also be fatigued. But the element that both share is a low glucose level within the cell, where the action is. Fatigue is a common symptom of many disorders, not just diabetes and hypoglycemia. Emotional factors (particularly depression), anemia, tuberculosis, and circulatory diseases are a few of the many other causes.

How is the low blood glucose produced? This can occur in many ways, but one of the simplest to explain is from an excessive production of insulin. This can result from an insulin-producing tumor in the pancreas. This, by the way, is a relatively rare medical problem. It acts just as if you had taken a needle and injected a lot of insulin into the body. All this insulin is capable of markedly lowering the blood-glucose level. Insulin shock and coma can result. Some tumors use large amounts of the blood glucose, causing rapid falls in the blood sugar. This too is an exceptionally rare problem.

Although physical exhaustion is often blamed as a cause of low blood glucose, in my experience it has been a relatively rare cause. Even in studies of pilots undergoing survival training and exhaustion who subsequently experienced fainting episodes, low blood glucose was seldom an important factor. It is true that physical activity increases the use of glucose and will tend to lower the blood level. But the simple truth is the body has a lot of reserve it can call upon before these mechanisms will cause seriously low blood-glucose levels in healthy people. The use of stored glycogen in the liver and muscles, the conversion of proteins to glucose, and even the use of fat for energy are all important mechanisms in combating low blood glucose resulting from just plain physical activity.

Lack of food intake as a cause for low blood sugar does occur in transitory states in some susceptible people, but even in prolonged starvation the blood-glucose level will normally be maintained at sufficiently high levels to prevent symptoms for long periods of time. You need only remember that people have been lost in the Arctic without food for seven weeks to recognize the truth of this observation. A lack of food intake becomes a significant factor in causing low blood glucose when it's associated with a change in daily habit pattern. I have in mind the person who is accustomed to eating breakfast and then suddenly stops the habit. He may indeed have symptoms attributable to low blood glucose for a few days until he has adjusted to a change in his habit pattern.

Remember that the liver is the glucostat. It can mobilize glycogen to pour glucose into the bloodstream and it processes glucose, fructose, and galactose. Whenever the liver is severely damaged it may have difficulty in responding normally and maintaining adequate blood-glucose levels. In rare hereditary conditions certain enzymes are missing that permit the use of some of the carbohydrates. For example, if a person with this exceptionally rare condition should ingest a small amount of fructose, it may cause a serious fall in the blood-glucose level.

Perhaps one of the most interesting causes of low blood glucose related to eating habits belongs to the general category of the dumping syndrome. In its full-blown manifestation this refers to reactions sometimes seen after a major portion of the stomach is removed, in treatment of an ulcer, for example. Normally the stomach acts as a food reservoir and gradually rations out the processed food into the small intestine. When the stomach isn't big enough to do this, all this food is rapidly dumped into the small intestine whether or not it is adequately processed. This will permit the accumulation of fluid with a high concentration of glucose in the small intestine, stimulating the release of hormones from the intestine that in turn stimulate the pancreas to pour out large amounts of insulin. As a consequence, low blood glucose, with the gamut of its symptoms, can follow.

Now not many people have had a major portion of their stomach removed to produce this problem, but many individuals have eating habits that can induce a small version of this problem. The person who has a rich carbohydrate breakfast, for example pancakes topped with syrup, followed by a cup of hot coffee loaded with sugar, is a candidate for this problem. The hot, sweet material from the coffee rapidly enters the small intestine. It's true that it can be absorbed only at a slow rate because the absorption is regulated by the intestinal wall itself. Even so, the concentrated glucose solution in the small intestine through hormone stimulation causes the release of large amounts of insulin. This mechanism is the same as in the genuine dumping syndrome.

This is particularly apt to occur at breakfast because the empty stomach will facilitate the rapid movement of hot, sweet liquids into the small intestine. It doesn't take the fasting stomach very long to process foods like hot cakes topped with syrup and other breakfast items that contain high concentrations of refined carbohydrates. When this problem is definitely the cause of low-blood-glucose symptoms, it can usually be modified by changing one's dietary habits. Incidentally, this is a good example of what is sometimes called reactive hypoglycemia. These persons will have normal fasting blood-glucose levels when they get up. The low blood-glucose level occurs as a reaction to the meal. This type of reaction is closely related to a condition sometimes called functional hypoglycemia in which the individual will have a low blood-glucose level three to four hours after carbohydrate ingestion.

Persons who are prone to diabetes may also have a reactive type of low blood glucose. Whenever they have a large amount of glucose in the small intestine it stimulates the release of insulin from the pancreas. Because of defects in the mechanism the release of the insulin is delayed too long. As a result, when insulin finally enters the bloodstream, the blood-glucose level is already diminished considerably by the use of glucose through other mechanisms. Consequently, the late insulin causes the blood-glucose level to fall too low and may induce symptoms. Reactive hypoglycemia related to the dumping syndrome, functional hypoglycemia, and the defective mechanisms of the patient prone to diabetes are often described as rebound low blood-sugar reactions. The theory behind the description is that as the blood-sugar level rises sharply, it induces overproduction of insulin which eventually causes the blood-glucose level to fall too low.

Among other rare causes of low blood glucose is failure of the pituitary gland to pour out its hormone which is antagonistic to insulin. Without the pituitary hormone, the balance relationship between it and insulin is disturbed, and this can cause attacks of low blood glucose. A tumor on the pituitary gland would be one reason for failure to pour out its special hormone.

Disease of the adrenal gland limits its effects in promoting the conversion of amino acids to glucose and other anti-insulin actions. It is also associated with low blood-glucose levels. But this condition, too, is relatively rare.

The question remains, what can one do about problems of low blood glucose? Remember, it's a finding, not a diagnosis; and of course the first thing to do is to verify the finding, and that means a competent medical examination. This includes a glucose tolerance examination. If the fasting blood-glucose level is normal, this rules out a number of conditions that may cause low blood sugar. If the low blood-glucose level, with attendant symptoms, occurs much later, after the glucose water has been administered, then it belongs in the reactive types of hypoglycemia.

It is necessary to make an accurate diagnosis of the cause of low blood glucose. If it is associated with a tumor of the pancreas, for example, the tumor should be removed. To cite another example, if it's caused by a specific enzyme failure associated with fructose, then the proper treatment would be to eliminate fructose from the diet, and that would include a lot of things, notably ordinary table sugar. If all the other causes can be eliminated and one is concerned principally about functional hypoglycemia, certain general diet principles seem to help. First, it's important to eliminate all concentrated sweets—table sugar, honey, syrups, jams, jellies, and similar foods. It's probably also wise to eliminate concentrated starches. Remember that starch is really packages of glucose, and once it gets into the small intestine it becomes glucose. The purpose of eliminating concentrated sweets and concentrated starches is to avoid the overconcentration of glucose in the small intestine which leads to a reactive type of low blood glucose. You can and should still have carbohydrate in the diet, but the carbohydrate should come from bulk foods such as leafy vegetables. If the diet contains sufficient bulk to delay the emptying of the stomach, it will help prevent having a concentrated solution of glucose in the small intestine with the undesirable reactive response. Remember that your aim here is to delay the emptying of the stomach and that means bulk foods are needed.

To illustrate one of the other changes you can make, it would be preferable to use tomatoes to obtain vitamin C than some of the fruits that contain reasonable amounts of sugar. Whole cereal can still be used in most people's diets, although how severe these restrictions are will depend on how severe the condition is. Many foods can be eaten even though a person has reactive hypoglycemia as long as they are eaten in the right sequence.

Remember that the emptying of the stomach is slowed with fat. It also empties slower with protein. Neither fat nor protein will increase the concentration of glucose in the small intestine. For this reason the person who has reactive hypoglycemia should use foods that are high in protein and fat and relatively low in carbohydrate. It would be better to eat the protein and fat foods first, followed by the carbohydrate, or at least to mix them together. If you are going to use a whole-wheat bread that would contain adequate amounts of cereal, you would be wise to eat it with meat and bulky vegetables.

Still another solution to delaying the emptying into the small intestine is to eat frequent very small meals. If the meals are small enough, this alone will help to delay the amount of glucose material which can arrive in the small intestine. Also, if you are going to eat fruit it would be wise to have it at the end of the meal so it can be mixed with the rest of the food items, diluting the glucose content with protein and fat.

The person with reactive hypoglycemia should follow some other food hints. One of these is to be absolutely certain to avoid hot, sweet liquids, particularly on an empty stomach. Remember that liquids tend to go straight through the stomach and into the duodenum. For this reason a hot cup of coffee loaded with sugar in the morning is particularly conducive to reactive hypoglycemia. Milk is not a bad choice but, even so, it contains a reasonable amount of carbohydrate. You need to have calcium in your diet, but you can accomplish this by substituting cottage cheese. It's a good source of quality protein and calcium, and much lower in carbohydrate content than milk. Over 25 per cent of the calories in whole milk are from carbohydrate, whereas in creamed cottage cheese only about 10 per cent of the calories are from carbohydrate.

As I mentioned, breakfast is probably one of the greatest challenges for the individual who has reactive hypoglycemia because then the stomach is empty. This means a change in breakfast patterns. If one wants to avoid the problem of ingesting too much fat, he can use fish for breakfast. It can be fried. Salmon patties can be used. For the rest of the day you can still have a diet that helps prevent reactive hypoglycemia without being too high in fat and cholesterol. You can accomplish this by using lean poultry and fish rotated with lean beef. The individual who has functional hypoglycemia can make life much more pleasant by readjusting what he eats, the order in which the foods are eaten, and how frequently he eats. If the problem is something other than hypoglycemia, these measures may appear to be helpful at first, as often happens with a variety of treatments for various medical problems. But in the long run the dietary management will not be successful, and a further search for other possible causes of the symptoms would certainly be required.

18

YOUR ENERGY SYSTEM NEEDS VITAMINS

Although vitamins contain no calories, they do generate a lot of heat—heated controversies between those for and those against. Judging from the number of individuals with a variety of qualifications, or lack of them, who proclaim themselves experts in this area, it is a game anyone can play. No wonder the public is generally confused about vitamins.

A large number of self-appointed vitamin gurus claim the way to health is to take large amounts of vitamins. If you listen to these individuals you would think that vitamins were high-energy compounds; in fact, they contain no calories. This means your body does not obtain any energy whatsoever from vitamins. Vitamins are substances our bodies require for their normal metabolic functions but cannot manufacture. In most instances, we obtain these vitamins from our food, although a principal source of vitamin D in sunny parts of the world is from the action of sunshine on chemicals in our skin. In addition, there are a group of substances called provitamins which are merely the substances from which vitamins are manufactured. A good example is beta-carotene, the yellow-pigmented provitamin the body processes to form vitamin A.

The relation of vitamins to the metabolic process is best explained by analogy. They are used in enzymes and coenzymes necessary to process energy foods, carbohydrates, fats, proteins, and alcohol. The energy is in these foods, not in vitamins. The enzymes, coenzymes, and their vitamin components are like the battery and electrical system on a car. The battery is necessary to start the engine, but it does not provide the engine's energy or horsepower. The energy comes from the fuel. When the engine is running, it recharges the battery. So it is with the enzymes, coenzymes, and vitamins—they are used to stimulate the process, and many are replaced by the metabolic process (the recharging phase). You will recall that the coenzyme NAD, containing the vitamin niacin, is used to carry hydrogen. It is returned to its usable stage (recharged) by stripping off the hydrogen which unites with oxygen to form water through the metabolic process. NAD is then ready to be used again.

Just as the horsepower of a car cannot be improved by adding two or three batteries to the engine, adding additional vitamins won't increase your energy level unless you have a vitamin deficiency in the first place. By analogy, an additional battery won't help your car run unless your battery isn't any good. But if your battery is down, the garage starts it with cables from a starter battery. So, if your car has a good battery, or if you have enough vitamins in your food—don't expect improved performance by more batteries or more vitamins.

Vitamin deficiencies are caused in several ways. The major ones are:

1. Inadequate ingestion of vitamins
2. Inadequate absorption of vitamins
3. Inadequate ability to use vitamins in the body
4. An increased requirement for vitamins (for example, in pregnancy)
5. Increased loss of vitamins in the urine or from the bowel
6. Any combination of these problems.

As you will see from the discussions of the individual vitamins, many of them are very important in accomplishing the metabolic processes. Without them the important enzyme and coenzyme systems that enable the cells throughout the body to strip the energy from our food could not work. There is a sound physiological basis for the observation that vitamin deficiencies can result in fatigue. Without adequate vitamins, our whole energy system is handicapped. Again, we see the importance of being able to extract energy from our foods if we want to avoid metabolic fatigue. This is true whether we're talking about delivery-of-oxygen problems, as can occur with anemia, or the absence of the basic calories to provide the energy, as occurs in a low-calorie diet, or the absence of vital substances such as vitamins that enable the foods to be processed.

There is still room for some controversy about how much of what vitamins the body needs. In many instances a decision has been made on the basis of being able to measure things, such as skin changes, anemia, or other objective physical changes that occur when there are not enough vitamins present. It seems reasonable to assume that other problems can occur before these more striking changes are readily apparent. It is not too great a strain on one's mental capacity to believe that one might experience some degree of fatigue because of disruption of our delicate energy mechanisms before gross anemia occurs, or before there are skin changes or other problems that can be photographed, measured, and quantified. Fatigue and energy levels are notoriously difficult to measure in a scientific way. What's worse, fatigue is caused by many other factors, including emotional problems, so it's very difficult to be objective about the cause of fatigue in any one case.

Even allowing for these observations, one can be relatively certain that the enormous doses advocated by some vitamin gurus serve no useful purpose. Once the tissues are saturated with a vitamin additional amounts are discarded through the urine, bowel, or combined systems. I like the analogy of pouring water into a cup. Once the cup is full, pouring in more water won't give you a bigger cupful. The body is the same way, and once you saturate it with a substance the rest is simply eliminated. When it's possible to measure this saturation point, as it is in a number of circumstances, we can at least set some outside limits beyond which additional amounts of vitamins are unlikely to provide any meaningful benefits.

The old concept of the Minimum Daily Requirement (MDR) has recently been replaced by the Recommended Daily Allowance (RDA) for nutrients. These figures are compiled regularly by the Food and Nutrition Board, National Academy of Sciences–National Research Council. The most recent revision, in 1973, is the basis for the values used here. The amounts they recommend are, in most cases, appreciably higher than the MDR values. In speaking of the significance of their values, the Food and Nutrition Board stated:

> The allowances are designed to afford a margin of suffi-
> ciency above average physiological requirements to cover
> variations among essentially all individuals in the general
> population. They provide a buffer against the increased
> needs during common stresses and permit full realization
> of growth and productive potential; but they are not to be
> considered adequate to meet additional requirements of
> persons depleted by disease or traumatic stresses. On the
> other hand, the allowances are generous with respect to
> temporary emergency feeding of large groups under con-
> ditions of limited food supply and physical disaster. The
> margin of safety above normal physiological requirements
> varies in extent for each nutrient. This occurs because of
> differences in the body's storage capacity, in the range of

individual requirements, in the provision of assessing requirements, and in the possible hazard of excessive intake of certain nutrients.

In other words, if you are healthy and your diet has sufficient nutrients to meet the RDA values for any or all vitamins, you will be getting sufficient amounts. Individuals who are ill or who already have a severe vitamin deficiency usually require larger amounts of vitamins for a period of time.

A healthy person eating an adequate, well-balanced diet of sufficient variety and amounts of all of the different foodstuffs will not have any vitamin deficiencies. The difficulty is that many individuals don't even understand what a well-balanced, normal, healthy diet should be. In addition, many other people are on fad diets, including recurrent fads for weight reduction, and for a variety of reasons aren't obtaining a good diet. Older people, particularly those who live alone, tend to eat diets that are not adequate in all respects. For this reason, vitamin deficiencies, at least to a minor degree, are much more common than need be, in view of the availability of food to most segments of the population in the industrialized nations. In short, vitamin deficiencies are more often a result of ignorance or lack of motivation than of availability.

Experimental work is underway using huge doses of vitamins, called megavitamin therapy, for certain medical conditions. This is a valid research area, but it has relatively little to do with the normal function of the normal body and the normal dietary intakes. These large doses are used with the idea that they serve as an actual medicine rather than as a nutrient. The Food and Drug Administration (FDA) has recommended that any dose of vitamins over one and a half times the RDA value must be considered as a drug or medicine rather than a nutrient. Even in medical problems, it's difficult to see how some vitamins can help when they are given in doses far in excess of what the body can hold or process. Let's take a case in point. It has been reported that taking more than 100 milligrams of vitamin C a day fails to cause any appreciable increase in blood concentration of vitamin C. It is difficult to see how much larger doses of vitamin C would result in delivering any increased amounts to the cells.

The value of megavitamin therapy will undoubtedly remain the subject of controversy for some time. It will be the arena for overly enthusiastic claims. This will have its adverse effects causing overly conservative and pessimistic reactions from the scientific community—comparable to what has become known in the political field as the backlash. Between the undisciplined enthusiasm of the faithful and the reactionary backlash group, there is still room for a good sensible approach to the amount of vitamins needed in the metabolic functions of the body. In my opinion, most of these are met by the RDA values when they are used in the context for which they were intended.

I must add to the consideration of vitamins for health my own amazement at the statements from the vitamin gurus. Adelle Davis was an outstanding contradiction. In one sentence she extolled the virtues of all that nutritious, lip-smacking, vitamin-rich Indiana farm food. It's what you eat and how you prepare it that makes the difference, she said. Then she advised popping down vitamin this and vitamin that. Some B for this and a lot of C for that. I don't think I need comment further on the inconsistency of such advice.

19

VITAMIN B₁, THIAMINE

Thiamine is the cereal vitamin. The illnesses caused by thiamine deficiencies were recognized long before the vitamin itself was identified. Perhaps one of the earliest observations of the problem was made by Admiral Takaki, who was Director General of Medical Services for the Japanese Navy in 1882. The Japanese sailors were existing on a diet of polished rice. He augmented their diet with meat, fish, and protein foods and eliminated the sailors' illnesses. It was a Dutch physician, however, who first recognized that many individuals on a polished rice diet were having problems because of the loss of a vital substance in the polishings. He prevented the problems of thiamine deficiency by adding rice polishings to the diet. To this day if cereals are processed so the husk is removed they will be deficient in thiamine. This is the reason white flour and other processed cereals are enriched with vitamin B_1.

It is not true, as often stated or implied by some vitamin gurus, that modern white bread and many of our cereals are deficient in the B vitamins. Regardless of what unattractive features one might be able to attribute to some of these products, notably white bread, all of these products are "enriched" with vitamins. In many instances these foods contain more vitamins than the original natural product, such as whole wheat. There is some danger that the practice of adding vitamins and minerals to bread and other products may become a hazard—there can be too much of a good thing. Our refined flour and white bread don't lack vitamins or minerals, but they may lack cereal fiber for needed bulk in the diet. Whether you prefer white bread, whole-wheat bread, or French bread, all are now enriched with vitamins and minerals.

Chemically, thiamine is a fairly complex structure. Despite this, it is constructed entirely of the building blocks of nitrogen, carbon, hydrogen, oxygen, and sulfur.

The presence of thiamine in the tissues is essential for their metabolic processes. Specifically, thiamine is a part of the enzyme system necessary for the conversion of pyruvic acid to active acetate. Remember that active acetate is a main metabolic intersection. In the absence of sufficient thiamine there is a buildup of pyruvic acid which in turn will mean an inability to process glucose or amino acids which are capable of conversion to glucose. A thiamine deficiency, then, affects carbohydrate metabolism. Thiamine is also essential to the body's ability to form the sugar ribose. Ribose is necessary to form the important RNA used in the cells to manufacture new proteins for all purposes within the body. Although perhaps of less vital importance to the metabolic processing system, thiamine is essential to form fatty acids.

Because thiamine is directly involved in the metabolic processing of carbohydrates, whenever a large portion of the calorie intake comes from carbohydrates the thiamine requirements are increased. Since cereals are carbohydrates, nature has wisely packaged thiamine in the natural cereal foods. Any factor that speeds up the metabolic requirements of the body, for example an overactive thyroid or even a normal pregnancy, also increases the need for thiamine.

A thiamine deficiency can produce a variety of symptoms which can progress to death. When reading these symptoms it is well to keep in mind that a lot of other factors produce many of these same symptoms. The difficulty of evaluating symptoms is pointed up by the problem of chest pain (not a symptom of thiamine deficiency). A heart attack can cause chest pains, but not all chest pains are heart attacks. Some may be muscular, others arthritic, pneumonia, or even problems within the esophagus. Symptoms alone do not make a diagnosis.

The classic form of a thiamine deficiency is referred to as beriberi. Among the disturbances it can cause are peripheral neuritis, tenderness along the course of the nerves, disturbances in the sensory sensations related to disturbed nerve function, and generalized nervousness often associated with poor concentration and poor memory. The pain and aching in the limbs associated with peripheral neuritis is one of the most striking complaints. Since metabolic actions go on throughout the cells in the body, it's not surprising that many parts of the body, including the heart, are affected by thiamine deficiency. In the presence of gross deficiencies heart failure can occur, the normal digestive functions are disturbed, sometimes causing a loss of appetite, and even the skeletal muscle's function is disturbed, leading to such problems as stiff neck and muscle soreness.

There is a limit to the thiamine the body can absorb. The most that can be absorbed is from 8 to 15 milligrams a day. Even this has to be accomplished by giving as much as 40 milligrams of thiamine in divided amounts, for example 10 milligrams four times a day. Any more than this taken by mouth will simply be eliminated through the bowels. More thiamine than this will have to be given by injection, circumventing the problem of absorption. An intake of 8 to 15 milligrams a day, however, is greatly in excess of the daily requirements.

Once the thiamine is absorbed it is distributed to all the tissues of the body. The highest concentrations are found in the liver, brain, kidney, and heart. When there is a large amount of thiamine in the diet, the tissues will become saturated with it. From that point on the body will destroy about one milligram of thiamine a day. This is the basis for the MDR of one milligram of thiamine. That's just enough to replace what the body destroys. When the intake is in excess of the MDR over a long period of time, the tissues will first become saturated. After that any excess amount above what the body needs to maintain this state will be eliminated in the urine. Thiamine is a water-soluble vitamin. After tissue saturation is achieved, additional intake will have no appreciable effects on the body except to increase the amount that is eliminated through the urine. The thiamine, then, ingested by persons who insist on taking huge daily doses of vitamins simply makes a rapid circuit through the body and out.

Using the current system of evaluating what the body needs in food items, the RDA for thiamine is relatively small.

Recommended Daily Allowance of Thiamine

Children	1–3 years	0.7 milligrams
	4–6 years	0.9
	7–10 years	1.2
Males	11–14 years	1.4
	15–22 years	1.5
	23–50 years	1.4
	over 50 years	1.2
Females	11–14 years	1.2
	15–18 years	1.1
	19–22 years	1.1
	over 22	1.0
	pregnancy	add 0.3
	lactation	add 0.3

The RDA values are not the most thiamine anyone should ever receive. If a person truly has a thiamine deficiency, as might be manifested by beriberi, then fairly large doses of thiamine are given initially until the tissues are saturated and the condition corrected. Once this is achieved, the above amounts based on the RDA should be sufficient.

The foods that most commonly contain appreciable amounts of thiamine are the cereals, peas, beans, lentils, soybeans, and nuts. There is also some in meat, milk, and other vegetables. The thiamine content in 3½ ounces (100 grams), edible portion, of common foods is:

Thiamine in Some Common Foods, per 100 Grams (3½ Ounces)

Almonds	.24 milligrams
Asparagus, raw spears	.18
Bacon, raw, cured	.36
Beans, mature seeds, raw, white	.65
red	.51
pinto	.84
lima	.48
Beans, green	.08
Beef, raw	.09
Beet greens	.10
Biscuits	.21
Bluefish	.12
Bran flakes (40 per cent bran), with added thiamine	.40
Brazil nuts	.96
Bread, enriched	.39
Cashew nuts	.43
Chicken	.06
Cornflakes, with added nutrients	.43
Corn, puffed, with added nutrients	.88
Cornmeal, whole-ground, unbolted	.38
degermed, enriched	.44
Cowpeas (black-eyed peas), immature seeds	.43
mature seeds	1.05
Dandelion greens	.19
Drum and Redfish	.15
Farina, enriched, regular	.44
Flounder and Sole	.05
Halibut	.07
Heart, beef	.53
calf	.63
hog	.43
Ham, separable lean, raw	.97
cooked	.64
Lamb	.15
Liver, beef	.25

Thiamine in Some Common Foods, per 100 Grams (3½ Ounces) (Cont.)

chicken	.19 milligrams
hog	.30
Macaroni, enriched	.88
Milk, whole	.03

(one cup, 8¾ ounces, 245 grams, contains .07 milligrams. A cup of milk fortified with 2 per cent nonfat milk solids contains .10 milligrams)

Noodles, egg, enriched	.88
Oatmeal, dry form	.60
Oranges	.10
Oysters	.13
Peanuts, raw with skins	1.14
Peas, green, immature seeds	.35
Peas and carrots, frozen, not thawed	.20
Pecans	.86
Pistachio nuts	.67
Pork, composite cuts	.81
Rice, brown	.34
white, enriched	.44
Soybeans, immature seeds	.44
mature seeds	1.10
Spaghetti, enriched	.88
Walnuts, black	.22
English or Persian	.33
Wheat flour, all-purpose, enriched	.63
Wheat bran, crude, commercially milled	.72
Wheat germ, crude, commercially milled	2.01
Wheat flakes, with added nutrients	.64
Wheat, shredded	.22
Yeast, Brewer's, debittered	15.61

The listed values for thiamine are based on the edible portion of the raw food unless otherwise stated. Cooking tends to destroy some of the thiamine. For this reason it's advisable to be generous in the use of items from this food list to be certain that sufficient thiamine is provided in the diet.

20

VITAMIN B₂, RIBOFLAVIN

Riboflavin is a pigmented vitamin. It was first identified in milk in 1879 and first called lactochrome because of its yellow color. Despite the complexity of the way it's assembled it is composed entirely of the building blocks of carbon, hydrogen, oxygen, and nitrogen.

Riboflavin is essential to use oxygen in the metabolic processing system. It is part of the "hydrogen express" and is the flavin unit in the system used to transfer hydrogen along the chain until it is combined with oxygen. Basically, then, it's involved in transporting the hydrogen that's picked up by the NAD and NADP coenzymes. Without this system it would not be possible to use oxygen and produce energy within the cells.

Considering the important role the flavins play in the metabolic process, it's surprising that a riboflavin deficiency doesn't cause more widespread damage than it apparently does in man. Most of the problems that have been described involve the body's surfaces. The mucous membranes around the mouth and lips may become inflamed, cracked, and crusted. There may be inflammations over the scrotum or the vulva area; the skin around the nose, ears, and eyes may become reddened, scaly, and greasy. Worst of all, the clear cornea of the eye that covers the pupil can gradually develop blood vessels in it and damage vision. There have been some reports of severe anemia in induced riboflavin deficiency in cancer patients which was corrected by replacement of riboflavin. All of these superficial manifestations, though, fail to tell us what the impact of a riboflavin deficiency could be on the energy system. Energy levels and fatigue do not show themselves objectively to be measured in centimeters or milligrams, or photographed for a demonstration. No doubt the importance of riboflavin in our diet and energy system is far greater than might be suspected by the paucity of symptoms that have been attributed to it.

Riboflavin is readily absorbed from the digestive tract and dispersed to all parts of the body. Very little of it, however, is stored in the tissues. The greatest concentration is stored in the kidney, the liver, and the heart. The failure to store large amounts of riboflavin means that adequate sources must be included regularly in the diet since there won't be any large tissue reserves to draw upon. Any excess riboflavin is eliminated in the urine.

How much riboflavin do you need? This varies with how many calories you are eating. The RDA values are:

Recommended Daily Allowance of Riboflavin

Children	1–3 years	0.8 milligrams
	4–6 years	1.1
	7–10 years	1.2
Males	11–14 years	1.5
	15–22 years	1.8
	23–50 years	1.6
	over 50 years	1.5
Females	11–14 years	1.3
	15–22 years	1.4
	23–50 years	1.2
	over 50 years	1.1
	pregnancy	add 0.3
	lactation	add 0.5

Riboflavin is not significantly affected by heat or cooking but it is very susceptible to light. As a result, you'll lose more vitamin B₂ from milk left on the doorstep than you will from its being pasteurized. A bottle of milk standing on the steps in the sunlight for only two hours will lose 85 per cent of its riboflavin.

Riboflavin is abundant in our food sources, and if you have a reasonable diet at all it's difficult to avoid getting sufficient amounts of it. A riboflavin deficiency is usually associated with other vitamin deficiencies since you have to eliminate so many foods to cause it. Riboflavin is commonly present in meat, milk, and cereals.

Riboflavin in Some Common Foods, per 100 Grams
(3½ Ounces) (uncooked edible portion)

Almonds	.92 milligrams
Bacon, Canadian	.22
Beans, white, red, pinto, mature seeds	.22
Beef, round steak, choice	.18
Biscuits	.21
Bread, enriched	.24

Riboflavin in Some Common Foods, per 100 Grams
(3½ Ounces) (uncooked edible portion) (Cont.)

Broccoli, raw	.23 milligrams
Cashew nuts	.25
Cheese, cheddar	.46
Cheese, cottage, creamed	.25
uncreamed	.28
Chicken, fryers	.23
Collards	.31
Dandelion greens	.26
Eggs (two)	.30
Farina, enriched, regular	.26
Heart, beef	.88
calf	1.05
hog	1.24
Herring, kippered	.28
Kidneys, beef	2.55
Lamb, composite cuts	.21
Liver, beef	3.26
calf	2.72
chicken	2.49
hog	3.03
turkey	1.93
Macaroni, enriched	.37
Milk, whole (times 2.5 for a cup)	.17
skim (times 2.5 for a cup)	.18
Mustard greens	.22
Noodles, egg, enriched	.38
Pancreas (sweetbreads)	.55
Pompano	.22
Pork, composite cuts	.17
Sausage, bologna	.22
Frankfurters	.20
Salami	.25
Shad, raw	.24
Spaghetti, enriched	.37
Spinach, raw	.20
Turnip greens	.39
Veal	.22
Wheat flour, all-purpose, enriched	.40
Yeast, Brewer's, debittered	4.28

21

NIACIN

Although the history of niacin is somewhat confusing, it is best known for its relationship to the dreaded condition of pellagra. Niacin belongs to the vitamin-B-complex group and like them is a water-soluble vitamin. Niacin deficiencies causing pellagra were once widespread throughout the southern United States. It is often associated with groups who depend heavily on corn and corn products as a major source of nutrition.

Niacin plays a very important role in the metabolic process. It, or the related substance nicotinamide, is part of the two essential coenzymes NAD and NADP. Remember, these are the coenzymes essential in transporting hydrogen in the metabolic process. By NAD enabling the transport of hydrogen to join oxygen, energy is released to form the high-energy ATP substances essential for the body's functions. It's no wonder then that niacin is essential to normal body function. NADP is essential in forming fatty acids for normal fat storage.

Chemically, niacin is a fairly simple substance. Its arrangement is rather complex but not nearly so complex as some of the other vitamin substances, and it's a fairly small unit. It, like many of the other vitamins, is composed only of blocks of carbon, oxygen, hydrogen, and nitrogen.

There's an interesting wrinkle to our body's need for niacin. We are able to manufacture it from the amino acid tryptophan. As you can see from this statement, our definition of a vitamin isn't too exact. Sixty milligrams of tryptophan can be converted into one milligram of niacin. Tryptophan is present in foods rich in high-quality proteins. The basis for developing pellagra (niacin deficiency) on a corn diet is explained by the conversion of tryptophan to niacin. The protein in corn is very low in tryptophan. If the direct sources of niacin are relatively limited, pellagra will occur if corn is the mainstay of the diet. In a diet containing protein with abundant amounts of the amino acid tryptophan, the tryptophan will be used to make niacin and pellagra will be prevented. Individuals using wheat, for example, are less likely to develop pellagra because the wheat protein contains appreciable amounts of tryptophan.

Pellagra induces a large range of symptoms of variable severity. It affects the skin, the digestive tract, and the nervous system. The mucous membranes which line the mouth and the lining of the entire digestive tract will become inflamed. This can cause watery, even bloody, stools. It's fair to say that the function of the entire digestive tract is out of kilter. Nausea, vomiting, and generalized symptoms related to the digestive tract are common.

Nervous system involvement causes headaches, dizziness, inability to sleep, mental depressions, delusions, hallucinations, and deterioration of total mental functions with personality changes. Normal movements and sensations may also be affected. Closely related to this is the "burning sensation" that many victims of pellagra complain of. Commonly there is severe anemia, perhaps related to a general slowdown in the metabolic functions of the body.

The skin changes most often involve the area exposed to the sun. As a result, a series of spotlike changes occur around the collar area at the base of the neck, much like a necklace. The inflamed, reddened skin areas tend to crop out in the springtime when exposure to the sunlight is increased.

In addition to these more definite symptoms of niacin deficiency, there remains the energy-fatigue area which is not so easily measured. Niacin has an essential role as part of the coenzyme systems NAD and NADP in the energy system in every cell in the body. It would be most unusual if a less than adequate intake of niacin, or its equivalent in tryptophan, did not result in generalized symptoms of fatigue and loss of energy.

Niacin is readily absorbed from the digestive tract, and because of its essential nature in the coenzyme system for metabolic functions, it is distributed throughout the cells in the body. Can you take too much niacin? Within reason, probably not. Any excess amount is rapidly eliminated through the kidneys. As such, excessive ingestion does not appear to cause any bodily harm. What you don't need, you lose.

Some doctors do prescribe very large doses—3000 to 6000 milligrams, in divided amounts, a day—to try to lower blood cholesterol levels, and sometimes it is helpful. These amounts are far in excess of any reasonable amount you might be taking on your own. Such megavitamin doses of nicotinic acid can cause problems, and anyone taking these amounts must be under a doctor's supervision. In these amounts it can cause severe skin flushing (usually temporary) and irritation of the stomach and rectum (probably irritation of the entire digestive tract) and interferes with the normal liver functions, even to the point of causing jaundice. This list of problems should make it clear why you should not be experimenting with megavitamin doses of even the B vitamins on your own. That liver damage can be serious. As you will see, however, these amounts of nicotinic acid, used as a medicine, are hundreds of times the amounts needed for your daily requirements for health.

The daily requirement varies a great deal depending on the quality of the diet, specifically, how much high-quality protein containing adequate amounts of tryptophan is included as well as natural sources of niacin. Foods important in providing niacin include liver, meat, poultry, and legumes. Milk and eggs are low in niacin, but their protein is fairly high in tryptophan so in this regard they are helpful. The niacin in cereals is most commonly in the husks, and is removed in any of the milling processes that eliminate the husks. Unfortunately, in many situations the niacin in the husks is not freed in our digestive process. In those circumstances it won't help us. It can be freed by preparing the food with an alkali. Such a process is commonly used in making tortillas, which explains why a properly made native tortilla can provide niacin.

The RDA values for niacin content or its equivalent in sufficient tryptophan are:

Recommended Daily Allowance of Niacin

Children	1–3 years	9 milligrams
	4–6 years	12
	7–10 years	16
Males	11–14 years	18
	15–22 years	20
	23–50 years	18
	over 50 years	16
Females	11–14 years	16
	15–22 years	14
	23–50 years	13
	over 50 years	12
	pregnancy	add 2
	lactation	add 4

The amount of niacin or niacin equivalent (60 milligrams of tryptophan for one milligram of niacin) in 3½ ounces (100 grams) of the uncooked, edible portions of common foods is:

Niacin in Some Common Foods, per 100 Grams
(3½ Ounces) (uncooked edible portion)

Almonds	3.5 milligrams
Asparagus spears	1.5
Bacon, cured	5.2
Bacon, Canadian	4.7
Bass	2.1
Beans, white, red, pinto, mature seeds	2.3
lima, mature seeds	1.9
Beef, round steak, choice	4.8
hamburger, lean	5.0
Biscuits	1.8
Bran flakes (40 per cent bran), with added thiamine	6.2
Bread	3.5
Cashew nuts	1.8
Catfish	1.7
Chicken, fryers	5.6
hens and cocks	9.2
Cod	2.2
Collards	1.7
Corn, sweet	1.7
Cornflakes, with added nutrients	2.1
Cornmeal, whole-ground, unbolted	2.0
Croaker	5.5
Drum and Redfish	3.5
Farina, enriched, regular	3.5
Flounder and Sole	1.7
Haddock	3.0
Halibut	8.3
Heart, beef	7.5
Lamb, composite cuts, choice	4.8
Liver, beef	13.6
chicken	10.8
hog	16.4
Macaroni, enriched	6.0
Noodles, egg, enriched	6.0
Oysters	2.5
Pancreas (sweetbreads)	5.8
Peanuts, with skins	17.2
without skins	15.8
Peanut butter	14.7
Peas, green	2.9

Niacin in Some Common Foods, per 100 Grams
(3½ Ounces) (uncooked edible portion) (Cont.)

Pork, composite cuts	4.1 milligrams
Potatoes	1.5
Rice, brown	4.7
white, enriched	3.5
Sausage, bologna	2.6
frankfurters	2.7
salami	5.3
Soybeans, mature seeds	2.2
Spaghetti, enriched	6.0
Tuna, canned, solids and liquids	10.1
Wheat flour, all-purpose, enriched	5.2
Wheat flakes, with added nutrients	4.9
Wheat, shredded	4.4
Yeast, Brewer's, debittered	37.9

22

PANTOTHENIC ACID

Pantothenic acid is a vitamin discovered in the early 1930s as a substance essential to the growth of yeast. The word comes from Greek and means "from everywhere," which amply describes the wide distribution of this substance in all the various foodstuffs.

Perhaps the most important aspect of pantothenic acid is its incorporation into Co-A. As you'll recall, Co-A combines with acetate to form active acetate, one of the most important metabolic crossroads where the glucose, fat, alcohol, and protein metabolic routes converge. Without question Co-A, and therefore its component, pantothenic acid, is absolutely essential to metabolics and providing energy for the body. A unit of pantothenic acid is fairly complex. Like many other organic units involved in our body and energy system, it is composed only of the building blocks of carbon, hydrogen, oxygen, and nitrogen.

A host of claims related to pantothenic acid have been made that are completely lacking in any scientific support by any valid research observations. There has never been a defined medical disorder in man from a deficiency in pantothenic acid, perhaps because of its widespread occurrence in food. A deficiency of pantothenic acid has been produced in animals, but the metabolic system of animals and man have important differences which are nowhere more apparent than in relation to some of the vitamins. In animals, pantothenic-acid deficiency can lead to degeneration of muscles and nerves, and even depress the function of the important adrenal cortex hormone gland to the point of causing death. The only indication of pantothenic-acid deficiency in man has been produced by formulating a diet devoid of pantothenic acid and then adding to the diet a chemical substance which destroys pantothenic acid (such substances are called antivitamins). This is an entirely artificial procedure. Taking a substance that destroys pantothenic acid would obviously destroy any amount normally available in the body, regardless of its source. This kind of experiment does not in any way establish the presence of a pantothenic-acid deficiency in man. Nevertheless, in using this combined procedure, symptoms of fatigue, headache, disturbed sleep, digestive disturbances, and muscle cramps have been described.

It's not surprising that a pantothenic-acid deficiency might produce fatigue. Without sufficient amounts it would be difficult for the normal metabolic processing system to produce adequate amounts of energy to run the ATP and energy-shuttle system for the body. And, as I mentioned before, it's relatively difficult to measure objectively changes in energy level or sensations of fatigue—a problem which plagues all vitamin research.

It is generally agreed that if the diet contains as much as 10 milligrams daily, that will be enough to satisfy our needs. Considering the widespread occurrence of the vitamin, there shouldn't be any difficulty in obtaining this much if the diet is adequate to meet other vitamin and protein needs. The richest sources of pantothenic acid are organ meats and whole-grain cereal.

Pantothenic acid is readily absorbed from the digestive tract. It is spread through the body, obviously, because of the necessity for Co-A action within all the cells. Its highest concentration is in the liver, adrenal gland, heart, and kidneys. It is not stored in any excess quantity. This again points up the necessity for regular replenishment of supplies. Excess amounts are eliminated—about two-thirds through the urine and the remainder in the food residue.

There is no valid evidence that giving pantothenic acid has any medicinal value. Fantastic claims have been made regarding its use in rheumatoid arthritis (that's not surprising—there have been lots of quack claims for cures of arthritis), changes in the nerves associated with diabetes, and even psychotic mental states. None of these claims is based on sound observations. Pantothenic acid has often been used to try to treat the "burning feet" problem common in prisoners of war. Careful studies have demonstrated it has no value here, either. The burning-feet problem is more likely related to other vitamin deficiencies.

The fantastic claims about pantothenic acid made in the public press by some vitamin gurus have led to many people taking pantothenic acid for problems it cannot help. Often these problems could be helped with competent medical supervision. This is the tragedy caused by vitamin gurus—they often induce people with real medical problems, who could benefit from competent diagnosis and treatment, to follow the futile hope of a miraculous cure from a vitamin. There is no better example of this than the use of pantothenic acid in the treatment of rheumatoid arthritis. Such patients deserve the complete and full attention of a specialist in rheumatoid arthritis problems, not another handful of pantothenic acid.

23

VITAMIN B₆, PYRIDOXINE

Pyridoxine is another vitamin that influences the condition of the skin and complexion. Pyridoxine was recognized by observing the skin disorders caused by a deficiency in rats. It is also another of those complex chemical compounds built out of the relatively simple blocks of carbon, hydrogen, oxygen, and nitrogen.

Pyridoxine is not as directly involved in metabolic functions as some of the other members of the vitamin-B-complex group. It is important, however, in the coenzyme systems responsible for the metabolic transformations of amino acids. It appears to be important in transferring amino blocks (nitrogen and two hydrogen blocks) to and from carbon skeletons. It also plays a role in removing individual carbon blocks (technically known as decarboxylation). Pyridoxine, then, is used within the amino-acid pool for transformations of amino acids. It is particularly important in the metabolism of tryptophan, the amino acid related to the melanin pigments in the skin, among other things.

Natural deficiencies of pyridoxine are rare in man. Disorders of the skin have been demonstrated by the artificial technique of using an anti-vitamin as well as a deficient diet. These include the oily seborrhealike skin changes prone to occur around the eyes, nose, and mouth. Inflammation of mucous membranes, particularly the lining of the mouth and the tongue, are apt to occur. In marked deficiencies even convulsions occur.

There is no evidence that even fairly large doses of pyridoxine are toxic in man. Really huge doses of 1 to 2 grams per pound of body weight (3 to 4 grams per kilogram) can cause convulsions and death in animals. Otherwise, there's no evidence of toxic reactions. The pyridoxine is rapidly absorbed from the digestive tract and then distributed widely throughout the body. It's not stored in any quantity in the body. This means a regular intake of pyridoxine is important to maintain adequate pyridoxine levels in the body.

Curiously enough, pyridoxine seems to exert a role in controlling the nausea and vomiting that occur in the early months of pregnancy, as well as the nausea and vomiting that sometimes follow radiation sickness. Rarely it seems to have a place in the treatment of certain anemias.

Pyridoxine is distributed widely in all kinds of food. Only a few foods are significantly lacking in it. The rich sources of it include meat, liver, vegetables, whole-grain cereals, and egg yolk. From this listing alone it's apparent that if a diet is adequate to meet the requirements for the other vitamins and protein intake, it's unlikely that a pyridoxine deficiency would occur.

The RDA values for pyridoxine for different age levels are:

Recommended Daily Allowance of Pyridoxine

Children	1–3 years	0.6 milligrams
	4–6 years	0.9
	7–10 years	1.2
Males	11–14 years	1.6
	15–18 years	1.8
	over 18 years	2.0
Females	11–14 years	1.6
	over 14 years	2.0
	pregnancy	2.5
	lactation	2.5

24

VITAMIN B₁₂, CYANOCOBALAMIN

Vitamin B_{12} is probably best known for its relation to pernicious anemia and liver extract. The absence of B_{12} goes far beyond its relationship to pernicious anemia. The anemia is a prominent feature only because our body produces the astonishing number of 200 million new red blood cells each minute. The mature, little, disclike red blood cells are without a nucleus, but they do have one in the early stages of their formation. The necessity to produce enormous numbers of new red blood cells on a minute-to-minute basis causes a deficiency of B_{12} to show up early by creating anemia. In areas of the body where the cell turnover is not so fast, the deficiency wouldn't be quite as noticeable that soon.

In a nutshell, the major role of B_{12} is to enable the vital DNA nucleic-acid strand within the cell nucleus to duplicate and separate. This is an essential process when one cell is giving birth to another cell—the process of biological regeneration. Each new cell must have DNA. Since this is essential to cell growth, it is clear that B_{12} is a growth factor. Without sufficient amounts of it, new cells can't be formed.

Vitamin B_{12} is also used in a coenzyme system involved in the changes occurring in the energy circle. Here its vital role is to enable energy formation by the breakdown of carbohydrates, proteins, fat, or even alcohol to run our biological system.

Chemically speaking, B_{12} is a very complex structure. It's a large unit, containing cobalt in addition to the carbon, nitrogen, oxygen, and hydrogen blocks common to most vitamins. B_{12} is ordinarily formed by microorganisms. Interestingly enough, a large amount of B_{12} is formed in our colon. We can't use it, however, because we don't absorb vitamins from the colon. In the scheme of nature the eliminated food residue, with its large amounts of B_{12}, is added to the total life system of planet earth.

The B_{12} in our food sources is tied to a protein at the time it's ingested. It arrives in the stomach in this condition. There the acid pepsin secretion breaks the protein part into polypeptides, and the B_{12} is split off. The B_{12} then joins with a substance formed by the lining of the stomach called intrinsic factor. This is absolutely essential if we are to derive any major benefit from B_{12}. The intrinsic factor formed in the wall of the stomach depends on adequate stores of iron. The union of intrinsic factor and B_{12} makes it possible for the B_{12} to be absorbed through the intestinal wall. In its absence the B_{12} will whistle right on through the digestive system and be eliminated with the rest of the food residue. Once the intrinsic factor with the B_{12} arrives in the small intestine, it must be attached to the intestinal wall before it is absorbed. This requires calcium, although magnesium may be used as a partial substitute. As you can see, it's a fairly complex process just getting the B_{12} through our digestive system and into the bloodstream.

Many individuals have pernicious anemia because their stomachs do not produce intrinsic factor. This is often associated with a low hydrochloric acid content. The whole process requires not only normal stomach function but also the presence of iron and calcium.

Once the B_{12} is absorbed into the bloodstream it is rapidly distributed throughout the body to support important cell functions. A large amount is stored in the liver for the body's reserve. The body can store from 1 to 10 milligrams. It tends to be fairly stable in the body. Some of it does leave the liver in the bile stream into the small intestine, but most of this is reabsorbed. Many individuals take large amounts of B_{12} and, indeed, physicians frequently give B_{12} shots for a variety of reasons. It's fortunate there don't seem to be any toxic reactions to even relatively large doses of B_{12}.

The outstanding early characteristic of B_{12} deficiency is pernicious anemia. This can become quite severe. It causes pallor and fatigue accompanied by all the usual symptoms attributed to anemia. There are two ways, then, that B_{12} deficiency can cause a lack of energy. One is by the anemia it produces, causing a deficiency of oxygen delivery to the cells. Whenever there is not enough oxygen available, the normal energy system cannot function properly and we don't get the usual amount of energy from our food. In addition, in coenzymes B_{12} is used along the processing line of the energy circle to strip the energy out of the various foods taking this route. Deficiencies here again mean that the cellular system is not up to par in extracting the total amount of energy from the food.

Even though anemia is a striking feature of the disease, there are many other manifestations of failure in fundamental cell function. One of these is growth. Consequently, it affects all of the tissues. The lining of the digestive tract is constantly being regenerated, and in the absence of normal regenerative capacities it's not surprising that there are a number of digestive complaints. The tongue is often sore. The abnormal processing of hemoglobin pigment and disturbed red blood cell formation often lead to a lemon-yellow tint.

Mental changes, including psychoses, are common in individuals with severe B_{12} deficiencies. I hastily add that this accounts for only a small number of mental problems since the vast majority of them are caused by other things. In view of the oxygen-energy deficit and the problem in regeneration and DNA formation, it's not surprising if the highly sensitive cells of the brain and nervous system function poorly. Having said this, it's equally important to point out that there's no evidence that increasing the amount of B_{12} in the diet, even in large doses, will cure or even improve mental disorders unless they are actually caused by an underlying B_{12} deficiency.

Nerve tissue is particularly sensitive to lack of oxygen. The combined mechanisms involved in B_{12} deficiency strike the nervous system hard, including the spinal cord and nerves. Cell changes here can lead to certain types of paralysis and a variety of findings that the nerve specialist can demonstrate in examining such patients.

The RDA values for vitamin B_{12} are:

Recommended Daily Allowance of Vitamin B_{12}

1–3 years	1.0 micrograms
4–6 years	1.5
7–10 years	2.0
Over 10 years	3.0
Pregnancy	4.0
Lactation	4.0

Since pregnancy involves marked duplication and growth of cells requiring constant splitting and formation of DNA, it is the period of greatest need for B_{12}.

The vitamin-B_{12} source in food may be labeled as cobalamin, or cyanocobalamin, and you can use these numbers as a guide to how much B_{12} is in your diet.

Vitamin B_{12} in Some Common Foods, per 100 Grams (3½ Ounces)

Organ meats, lamb, beef liver, kidney, heart, clams, oysters	10 micrograms
Nonfat dry milk, crabs, rockfish salmon, sardines, egg yolk	3 to 10
Muscle meat, lobster, scallops, flounder, haddock, swordfish, tuna, and some cheeses	1 to 3
Whole milk	less than 1

25

FOLIC ACID AND PABA

Folic acid has a lot in common with vitamin B_{12}. It's also vital to cell growth, particularly the formation of DNA and RNA. It is a very complex arrangement of nineteen carbon blocks with blocks of hydrogen, nitrogen, and oxygen. Part of its structure includes PABA (para-aminobenzoic acid) and glutamic acid. Folic acid is also called folacin and belongs to a group of related chemicals called folates.

The main action of the folates is to form coenzymes important in transferring a block of carbon with attached hydrogen blocks to other compounds. Such transfers are important in forming purine and pyrimidine bases. You will recall that these compounds are the teeth in the long chain of those all-important nucleic acids, RNA and DNA.

A folic-acid deficiency causes an anemia that is indistinguishable from the pernicious anemia caused by B_{12} deficiency. Because both vitamins play a vital role in cell reproduction, both are necessary in producing those 200 million new red blood cells each minute.

Even though the anemia is the most striking effect of a folate deficiency, it isn't the only symptom. Throughout the body, where there is a constant turnover of cells, there is trouble. The tongue is sore. The constantly regenerating intestinal track is disturbed, resulting in diarrhea, weight loss, and a host of symptoms of indigestion.

Unlike a B_{12} deficiency, a folic-acid deficiency doesn't affect the spinal cord. One big difference, then, in the problems is that B_{12} deficiencies cause spinal-cord changes, often creating difficulty in walking, and folate deficiency does not. There is evidence of disturbed brain function, however. Victims often complain of forgetfulness, insomnia, and irritability. But a lot of other problems cause those symptoms. It is possible that they are a result of the anemia's hindering delivery of oxygen to sensitive brain cells.

Folic acid is readily absorbed from the digestive tract. The synthetic pure form is used to better advantage by the body than is the natural vitamin because the natural form is bound to other compounds and is not as readily available for direct use. This, incidentally, gives the lie to the oft-repeated statement that natural vitamins are better than synthetic vitamins. About 0.1 microgram (one millionth of a gram or one thousandth of a milligram) of pure folic acid is equivalent to 0.4 microgram in food sources, and that meets the daily requirements except during pregnancy and lactation or periods of unusual physiological stress.

Any excess folic acid is readily eliminated through the kidneys. It is not toxic even in large doses. Nevertheless, the Food and Drug Administration has limited the amount that can be included in vitamin tablets to 0.1 microgram. This is for your safety. Larger doses of folic acid can correct the anemia of a B_{12} deficiency. As the B_{12} deficiency goes untreated, those changes start in the spinal cord. If the anemia weren't corrected by the folic acid, masking the B_{12} deficiency, the patient would go to a doctor and get the needed B_{12}.

The RDA values for folacin from food sources are determined by a technique using lactobacillus. The values are four times as great as the amount needed of the pure form of folic acid.

Recommended Daily Allowance of Folic Acid

1–3 years	100 micrograms
4–6 years	200
7–10 years	300
Over 10 years	400
Pregnancy	800
Lactation	600

Folic acid is present in many foods. It was isolated from spinach leaves, and because of its presence in foliage it was called folic acid. Liver is a rich source. You can also get a lot of it in leafy vegetables, other vegetables, and many types of fruit. There is also a reasonable amount in nuts, mature bean seeds, and peas. Large amounts of it are destroyed in cooking. You can see now why those fresh leafy salads are important in your diet. Other than its occurrence in liver, it is mostly a vitamin of the plant world. If you want to get your share of folic acid, don't forget to include plenty of fresh leafy vegetables—preferably raw—in your diet.

Despite certain wild claims about the virtues of PABA, it has no value in mammals. We can't use it to form folic acid. Some bacteria do use it in forming folic acid, and it is essential to these microorganisms. In fact this is how certain sulfa drugs work, by destroying the PABA in the bacteria and thereby destroying their ability to multiply. Remember, folic acid is important in the DNA-RNA system essential to cell growth and reproduction.

26

BIOTIN AND INOSITOL

Biotin is considered a vitamin and it's another of those complex chemical units made of building blocks of hydrogen, nitrogen, oxygen, and carbon. Biotin appears to play a fundamental role along the metabolic processing line by helping to attach carbon dioxide to other compounds. This is sometimes necessary in building carbon chains to form new compounds. It may also be important in supporting the removal of a carbon unit from OAA as it goes along the metabolic path to form active acetate.

In reading the voluminous information on food and health, you may have come across the statement that raw egg whites can be injurious. There is some basis of truth to this statement, and it's related to biotin. Don't worry about it, though, unless you are accustomed to eating raw egg whites.

The reason egg white tends to cause biotin deficiency is that it contains an antivitamin called avidin. It neutralizes the actions of biotin, leading to "egg-white injury." In fact, this is the way biotin was first discovered. Raw egg whites were fed to rats as the sole source of their protein. In the course of time they developed disorders of their muscles with inflammation of the skin and loss of hair. When the egg white is cooked, the avidin action is destroyed.

There has never been any evidence of spontaneous biotin deficiency in man. Experimental studies comparable to those done on the rat have been carried out in which a biotin-deficient diet was consumed along with large amounts of raw egg whites. In three to four weeks the skin became quite scaly.

Biotin doesn't seem to have any toxic actions. It is readily absorbed in the digestive tract and excess amounts are excreted in the urine.

How much biotin is required by man isn't known, since there has never been any evidence of deficiency of it. This again may be misleading since it's difficult to evaluate energy levels and fatigue. It's probable that biotin is so widespread in food that deficiencies of it are unlikely to occur in anyone receiving anywhere near an adequate diet. It is present in large amounts in yeast, liver, kidney, egg yolks, cauliflower, nuts, and legumes.

I am mentioning inositol only for completeness' sake and because Adelle Davis had championed it as having all sorts of health benefits. It is a growth factor in yeast and certain bacteria. If you were a mouse or a rat you might need it, at least to prevent loss of hair. And it is essential to the growth rate of hamsters, chicks, and guinea pigs. But guinea pigs we are not. Physiologists, reputable nutritionists, and biochemists have all failed to identify any defect in man related to inositol deficiency. Nor have they identified a single role of the substance in the metabolic process. I think you can safely forget about inositol.

27

VITAMIN C, ASCORBIC ACID

The colorful history of vitamin C includes the devastating episodes of scurvy that laid waste to the Crusaders, and the hot debate over its use in treating and preventing the common cold. Scurvy was apparently one of man's earliest scourges. Briefly, scurvy affects all of the connective tissue in the body, including the ligaments and the material that binds the cells together. It causes the teeth to become loose and the gums to be spongy with a tendency to bleed. There is a tendency throughout the body for easy hemorrhaging into the skin. In children scurvy damages the bone. As the disease progresses, its widespread effects on the body's connective tissue systems cause changes that result in death.

Many historians credit the defeat of the early Crusaders in the 1300s and 1400s to the prevalence of scurvy. The history of scurvy reaches to the early colonies of the United States and Canada. Scurvy became a sailor's disease when it became possible to build boats big enough and strong enough to remain at sea for long periods of time.

The relationship of scurvy to fresh fruits was recognized by 1600. About this time the ships of the East India Company used oranges and lemons to prevent scurvy. The use of lemons and limes by the British Navy to prevent scurvy is the basis for the slang term "limeys" applied to British sailors. Until fairly recently, man was unable to preserve fresh fruits high in vitamin C. During the cold winter months, people gradually became more and more deficient in vitamin C. As the warm weather returned, providing fruits and vegetables to remedy this condition, health was restored. This may well be the basis for the centuries-old concept of a "spring tonic."

The chemical compound of vitamin C was first isolated as late as 1932 and, surprisingly, it's very much like glucose. It has a six-carbon-chain skeleton and is made totally of carbon, oxygen, and hydrogen blocks. You can think of it diagrammatically as in Figure 37.

The similarities between vitamin C and glucose are no accident. Most

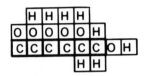

Fig. 37. Ascorbic acid (vitamin C).

animals are able to use glucose to form whatever amounts of vitamin C they need. But as I have repeatedly pointed out, man and animals do not have the same metabolic system. Within the animal kingdom, man, the other primates, and the guinea pig are the principal mammals unable to convert glucose to ascorbic acid. I can't resist pointing out that the vitamin gurus are fond of identifying a disorder in animals because of a vitamin deficiency and then claiming the same thing happens in man. This blatant disregard for the differences in the metabolic system of man and animals is responsible for a lot of misinformation given to the public. There is no better example of the difference than man's inability to make vitamin C. The other mammals contain an enzyme in the liver that enables the conversion of glucose to vitamin C.

All of this might suggest to the naturalist that man, like the other primates, developed in climates where abundant sources of vitamin C were naturally available. Since vitamin C is the component of plants which are chiefly carbohydrates, this again supports the concept that early man, like other primates, obtained a major portion of his food from vegetation, not from high fat–high protein sources as has been erroneously stated by such books as *Calories Don't Count* and *Dr. Atkins' Diet Revolution*.

Although vitamin C deficiency has been known for centuries, there are still a great many holes in our knowledge of how vitamin C affects our metabolic processing system. It is generally believed that it has some effects on the use of oxygen in producing energy, but exactly what these are we don't know. It also has some effects on metabolism of the amino acid tyrosine. Animals who are deficient in ascorbic acid—called scorbutic animals—appear to have a disturbance in their carbohydrate metabolism. They tend to develop high blood-glucose levels and are resistant to insulin. Vitamin C also plays some role in the changes of folic acid in the body.

The one recognized and generally agreed-on function of vitamin C in the body is its role in the formation of collagen. This is a substance in tissues that yields gelatin. The strandlike collagen material is the basis for developing the tiny membranes and connective tissue that hold together the muscle fibers and cells and is used around joint membranes and all other membranes that line the organs and body cavities. These substances bind together our blood vessels, our bones, and even the ligaments that hold our teeth tightly in place. Because of its important role in the formation of this connective tissue, adequate levels of vitamin C in the body are particularly important to wound-healing as well as prevention of scurvylike episodes.

You need to know what vitamin C does *not* do in the body. I well recall in my early years in medicine, before the powerful pituitary and adrenal steroid hormones were available, large doses of ascorbic acid were frequently used in many illnesses related to "stress." Basically, large doses of vitamin C were used as a substitute for adrenal hormone. Regardless of the other benefits of vitamin C, it is not a substitute for adrenal hormone. The high concentration of vitamin C in the adrenal gland led to this supposition, but it was nothing more than supposition. The practice of using vitamin C as a substitute for adrenal hormones has, of course, disappeared since these substances are now readily available.

Vitamin C is rapidly absorbed from the digestive tract. It is distributed in limited amounts throughout the body, with the highest concentration in glandular tissue. It is partially destroyed in the body. Vitamin C is not stored in the body, so your diet should include adequate amounts of vitamin C daily. When the intake exceeds the body's needs, it can be converted to a substance called oxalate for elimination in the urine. In large amounts this may be capable of producing kidney stones. Vitamin C is not eliminated in the urine unless the body is sufficiently saturated with it. This is an important concept; if you are pouring out a lot of vitamin C in the urine, your body already has all it needs.

How much vitamin C do you need? There are certainly a lot of hot debates on that. If your diet contains as much as 60 milligrams of vitamin C a day, that will meet the RAD for all age groups. At least this is true for nonsmokers. There is some evidence that smoking destroys vitamin C. One scientist claims smoking a single cigarette destroys as much vitamin C as you'll find in one orange. That's a lot of vitamin C. There are problems of losing vitamin C in food storage and preparation. You would be wise to obtain a major portion of your vitamin C from raw fresh fruits and vegetables. Otherwise you should have double or triple the usual amount of items listed to provide the 60 milligram RDA standard.

There are reports that taking more than 100 milligrams a day of vitamin C will not increase the amount of vitamin C in the blood. In other words, there is an upper ceiling as to how much vitamin C your blood can carry. If you consume more vitamin C than is necessary to reach this level, it is simply destroyed in the body or eliminated through the kidneys. These studies suggest, then, that a daily intake of beyond 100 milligrams of vitamin C serves no real purpose.

This concept is not shared by a number of vocal vitamin gurus. One of the more vocal of these, Irwin Stone, has long been one of the proponents of much larger doses. He and Linus Pauling claim that since primates in their natural habitat consume 4 or 5 grams of vitamin C a day, we too should be consuming much more. Linus Pauling suggests 2.3 grams per day. The enthusiasm of the massive-vitamin-intake proponents knows no bounds. Large doses of vitamin C have been credited with curing viral infections, bacterial infections, heart disease, arthritis, various forms of rheumatism, allergies, ulcers, diseases of the kidney and the bladder, diabetes, and a seemingly endless list of medical problems. The claims are reminiscent of the old-fashioned medicine-show techniques and sound similar to the recurrent themes of enthusiasts for miracle cures. Discerning physicians who have been actively participating in medicine for years recognize the symptoms. Time after time, when a new preparation appears or an old one is rediscovered, it suddenly develops magical qualities for everything from itch to idiocy. Such ill-founded enthusiasm has occurred with certain hormones that do have specified, but limited, uses and certainly with vitamins. You can hardly blame physicians for being at least moderately skeptical when enthusiastic claims are initially proposed, at least until adequate amounts of valid research have been achieved.

On the basis of the most recent wave of enthusiasm for vitamin C, daily doses of 1 to 4 grams have been recommended; and Linus Pauling claims that it is the long-sought cure for the common cold, among other all-encompassing benefits. To prevent colds he recommends that one take 2 grams of ascorbic acid a day. At the very first sign of a cold he recommends increasing this to 1 gram per hour until the symptoms have disappeared, and higher dosage than the usual daily amount for a few days thereafter to prevent a recurrence.

The controversy that has ensued has not been totally resolved. It's fair to say that most of the studies bearing on this issue to this date indicate that in large amounts, possibly 1 gram a day, even if colds are not prevented the severity of the disagreeable symptoms may at least be diminished. This, however, gets into the area that's difficult to quantitate. The value of the vitamin in aborting a cold or curing it once it has started has not received widespread enthusiastic endorsement. On the contrary, there have been numerous reports of less than spectacular results. The proponents of high vitamin C dosages have claimed that this is because the vitamin isn't given soon enough, and the cold has been allowed to establish itself. No doubt the controversy will continue to rage because it seems that neither the proponents nor the detractors choose to be confused with the facts. At present, though, it seems safe to say that the common cold isn't suddenly going to disappear from our midst merely from the use of large doses of vitamin C.

Moderate doses of vitamin C are completely nontoxic, and the excess amount is eliminated from the body. This does not apply to the huge doses advocated by some of the vitamin C proponents. As Linus Pauling acknowledges, the large doses of vitamin C he advocates can cause diarrhea because of its laxative effect. This is not totally an innocuous response in some individuals, particularly those who are prone to have digestive disorders. Russian studies have demonstrated that pregnant rats given large doses of vitamin C tend to have abortions; and among twenty pregnant women, sixteen developed menstrual-type bleeding when they were given vitamin C. The basis for this appears to be an increase in formation of the female hormone, estrogen, causing the uterus to be overactive. This at least should suggest caution to pregnant women about the unsupervised use of massive doses of vitamin C. Other adverse effects from large doses of vitamin C include reports of painful urination and, for the very large doses of 4 to 12 grams a day, the possibility of developing kidney stones.

What then should one do about one's daily dose of vitamin C? The evidence is so meager that more than one gram a day is of any help to anyone, it would seem logical that this is sufficient. Additional amounts even at the onset of an acute cold are not going to materially improve the situation. For this reason I do not recommend people dosing themselves in excess of one gram per day, and probably this should be divided into one-half gram in the morning and one-half gram in the evening.

Individuals who consume large amounts of fresh raw fruits and vegetables probably have no reason to concern themselves about their vitamin-C intake. You can waste a lot of effort concerning yourself about food preparation and storage for vitamin C because the main source in your diet should be fresh raw fruits and vegetables. Oranges, apples, grapefruit, and tomatoes are all good sources of vitamin C.

Vitamin C in Some Common Foods, per 100 Grams (3½ Ounces)

Broccoli, cooked	90 milligrams
Brussels sprouts, boiled, drained	87
Cabbage, cooked	33
raw	47
Cauliflower, raw	78
cooked	55
Collards, cooked	76
Grapefruit, raw, all varieties, composite value	38
Lemons, raw	53
Limes, raw	37
Muskmelons	33
Mustard greens, cooked	48
Mustard spinach, cooked	65
Oranges, composite, all varieties	50
Papaya	172
Pimientos, canned, solids and liquid	95
Tangerines	31
Tomatoes	23
Turnip greens, cooked	69

28

VITAMIN A

How the pendulum has swung in the course of time! Many years ago vitamin deficiencies were a world-wide problem. Now the danger in many of our industrialized nations is vitamin toxicity. This applies specifically to the fat-soluble vitamins such as vitamin A. So many of our foods are fortified and enriched that if vitamins really did contain a lot of energy they would be jumping off the shelves in the supermarkets. This, coupled with vitamin tablets containing large doses of such substances as vitamin A available to the public without prescription, has led to this new problem of developed nations.

Vitamin A is essential for normal growth. It is a fairly large unit, consisting of twenty carbon blocks, thirty hydrogen blocks, and one oxygen block. Nevertheless, it's just a straight carbon chain like the fatty acids. It has been converted to an alcohol through the simple expedient of adding one unit of water. Chemically then, it's not much different from a fatty acid.

One important area of confusion should be cleared up about the difference between carotene and vitamin A. Carotene is a provitamin, meaning that it can be used to make vitamin A. It is the yellow-pigmented substance present in carrots, other yellow vegetables, and green-pigmented vegetables. In the undigested state it's not usable by the body, but it can be split into two parts because it's essentially a double vitamin-A unit. Once it's split, only half of it can be used for vitamin A. Because of a minor variation in the way the blocks are put together, the other half cannot be used for vitamin A. In listing the amount of vitamin A in different food substances, most tables take this into account when they include vegetables rich in beta carotene as sources of vitamin A.

It's the carotene that provides the yellow pigmentation. Vitamin A is not yellow, but white. Until this was cleared up, it led to a great deal of confusion. Investigators looked for the yellow-pigmented material and were startled to find that some foods that weren't yellow seemed to be richer in vitamin A. In these foods the carotene had already been converted to vitamin A. This is the reason pale milk is often richer in vitamin A than yellow milk, and why pale natural butter may contain more real vitamin A than golden-yellow butter. Stated simply, yellow doesn't mean it's better.

Some animals are able to manufacture vitamin A in their body and store it in their liver and carcass. Carnivores, as a group, cannot manufacture vitamin A. They meet their vitamin-A requirement by eating the carcasses of animals that can.

Vitamin A influences the metabolic processing of carbohydrate indirectly through its role in the formation of adrenal-cortex hormones (technically called the glucocorticoids). Remember from the discussion about blood-glucose levels that the adrenal-cortex hormones tend to neutralize the effects of insulin, and so to raise blood-glucose levels. This indirect relationship of vitamin A to blood-glucose levels has given rise to enthusiasm for the possibility of using large doses of vitamin A to treat low blood glucose. However, this treatment would be effective only if the individual were deficient in vitamin A to begin with.

In line with its growth-stimulating function, and possible other effects on cell formation, vitamin A is essential to the formation of sperm. In vitamin-A deficiencies, male sterility, which can be permanent, may occur. A major role of vitamin A is in maintaining healthy surface cells. This includes all those cells which line the inner surfaces of our body, such as the lining inside the lungs and the digestive tract. It also affects the outer surfaces of the skin and particularly the eyes. The surfaces of the body, both inside and outside, are areas of rapid cellular replacement even after we become adults.

Still another function of vitamin A is the important role it plays in complex chemical changes in the back of the eye that improve the ability to see at night. The fact that carotene can be converted to vitamin A and that vitamin-A deficiencies have been associated with poor night vision has led to the observation that eating lots of carrots sometimes improves night vision. It will if you are deficient in vitamin A, but the claims that it will accomplish this within a few minutes are ridiculous. It takes considerably longer than that for the body to process carotene and convert it to vitamin A to correct vitamin A-deficiencies. Nevertheless, a regular intake of carrots, or any other source of carotene, or vitamin A itself will help to prevent this bad night vision.

Vitamin A is usually classified as a fat-soluble vitamin but it is not so dependent on fat for absorption through the digestive tract as was once thought. Actually, it's fairly rapidly absorbed from a water solution. The water-solution preparations of vitamin A are better than those that have been prepared with oil suspension. If you are in the habit of taking mineral oil regularly—which I don't advise—you should know that it will impede the absorption of vitamin A. Individuals who have particular problems in fat absorption, as may occur with pancreatic and gall bladder diseases, usually do better if they take vitamin A in a water solution, if they take it at all.

As just one of numerous examples of misinformation provided to the public about the use of vitamins, Adelle Davis had repeatedly stated that you must drink whole milk because you need the fat in the whole milk to absorb the vitamin A milk contains. In the first place, it's almost impossible to cause the diet to be grossly deficient in fat, as you should realize from the earlier discussion about the fat content of various foods. You have to make a real effort to have a fat deficiency, unless you have an underlying medical problem that affects absorption of fat. In the second place, fat isn't that essential to the absorption of vitamin A. In short, this statement is completely without scientific basis. There is no reason whatsoever to drink whole milk to assure the absorption of vitamin A from the digestive tract. Fortified skim milk products, uncreamed cottage cheese, and nonfat dry milk powder are all excellent foods, and the absence of fat in these products will not interfere with the absorption of vitamin A. All these and many other products available to us are fortified or enriched to provide us with vitamin A as well as to help us prevent atherosclerosis.

The absorption of vitamin A is enhanced by thyroid hormone. Persons with low thyroid functions have trouble absorbing it. This may explain why giving thyroid to men who have moderately low thyroid function greatly enhances their fertility. The thyroid enhances the absorption of vitamin A, and the vitamin A improves formation of sperm. Incidentally, improving or increasing the formation of sperm does not mean increasing the formation of the male hormone testosterone or otherwise affecting sexual performance.

Once the vitamin A is absorbed in the body, the major portion of it is stored in the liver. That's why liver is such a rich food source of vitamin A. Cod liver, and particularly halibut liver, are very rich in vitamin A. Eating large amounts of them can produce acute vitamin A toxicity. Eating polar bear liver, which is very rich in vitamin A, can cause a severe, acute illness, often leading to death.

As you might expect from the various roles of vitamin A, a deficiency in it will cause problems of growth in the young and will effect tissue replacement, such as the surface cells. There will be poor night vision and overgrowth of the gingiva (gums) around the teeth; the ability for reproduction may be adversely affected, and there may be an overgrowth of bone. Among the most common problems of prolonged vitamin-A deficiency are changes in the cells over the surfaces of the eye, causing reddening and sometimes leading to blindness. Severe vitamin-A deficiency is still a cause of blindness in many parts of Asia.

In our society vitamin-A deficiency is often blamed for changes in the skin, though it's seldom the underlying cause. Deficiencies of vitamin A will cause abnormal shedding of the old surface cells and other changes which make the skin more susceptible to infection. For this reason, vitamin-A deficiency is identified with acne or pimples. The common occurrence of acne in adolescence—related to the sudden outpouring of sex hormones—often leads teenagers into the ill-advised practice of taking huge doses of vitamin A. As a result, cases of vitamin-A toxicity have been seen with increasing frequency in recent years.

With moderate chronic vitamin-A toxicity, there is a time period between the onset of overdosage and the development of toxic reactions. Usually this time interval is about six months. The findings are variable, some of them even mimicking vitamin-A deficiency. Individuals suffering from this problem will be irritable, suffer loss of appetite, and sometimes complain of abdominal discomforts. They'll have skin problems too, usually itching, cracked and bleeding lips, and loss of hair. There are often tender deep swellings over bony prominences, such as over the back of the head, and eventually extra heavy bone deposits over certain areas. Because of other changes that affect fluid retention, there may be swelling in the brain. This will cause changes in the eye and symptoms closely resembling brain tumor.

Many a young person taking large doses of vitamin A over a long period of time has had a preliminary diagnosis of brain tumor until someone discovered his vitamin-popping habit, giving him a clue as to the real cause of the disorder. This should be warning enough for individuals who are tempted to use massive doses of vitamin A on their own. Fortunately, the toxic symptoms of vitamin A will usually disappear in about one week after vitamin A has been discontinued—provided someone discovers that's what's causing the problem. Reversal of the bony changes, however, takes much longer.

The sudden toxic reactions that can occur from ill-advised eating of halibut liver or polar bear liver cause a severe attack of nausea, vomiting, and stomach pain. Following the initial crisis, the skin will start peeling and continue for days or even weeks.

Considering the problems of deficiency and toxicity, just how much vitamin A should your diet include?

Recommended Daily Allowance of Vitamin A

1–3 years	2000 I.U.
4–6 years	2500
7–10 years	3300
Males over 10	5000
Females over 10	4000
Pregnancy	5000
Lactation	6000

There is no satisfactory evidence that taking more than 25,000 units a day will provide any additional benefit, even for vitamin-A deficiency. For an actual deficiency, dosages this high might be used. Once the tissues are saturated and the liver stores are replaced, it's better to stick to the RDA values. The continued taking of any amounts in excess of 25,000 units for long periods of time increases the risk of developing vitamin-A toxicity. This has led me to recommend to patients, regardless of their motivation for taking high doses of vitamin A, to stay under 25,000 units a day, including the vitamin A in food as well as that in vitamin pills. In most instances, there should be no reason for taking even this large amount for any extended period of time. For anyone not suffering a deficiency, if they are not pregnant or lactating, there is no valid reason for taking more than 5,000 units a day.

Look carefully at any vitamin pills you are taking and see how much vitamin A they contain. If you add this amount to the vitamin sources in the milk, cereals, bread, and other foods you need, you may be getting too much. The Food and Drug Administration has recommended restricting the sale of preparations containing more than 10,000 units of vitamin A to prescription items. This is because of the increased number of toxic cases, and because so much food is "enriched" with extra amounts.

As a guide for your food requirements for vitamin A, the values for vitamin A (carotene units have been converted to vitamin-A equivalents) are:

Vitamin A in Some Common Foods, per 100 Grams (3½ Ounces)

Apricots, raw	2700 I.U.
Broccoli, raw	2500
Butter	3300
Carrots, raw	11,000
cooked	10,500
Cheese, cheddar	1310
Cherries, red sour, raw	1000

Vitamin A in Some Common Foods, per 100 Grams (3½ Ounces) (Cont.)

Chives, raw	5800 I.U.
Collards, cooked	7800
Crab, steamed	2170
Cream, light whipping	1280
Cress, garden, raw	9300
Dandelion greens, cooked	11,700
Eggs, whole raw (2)	1180
Halibut, broiled	680
Lettuce, cos or romaine, looseleaf, raw	1900
Liver, beef, fried	53,400
calf, fried	32,700
chicken, fried	12,300
hog, fried	14,900
turkey, simmered	17,500
Mangoes, raw	4800
Margarine	3300
Milk, whole	1130
Muskmelon and Cantaloupe	3400
Mustard greens, cooked	5800
Mustard spinach	8200
Nectarines	1650
Papaya, raw	1750
Peaches, raw	1330
Peas and carrots, cooked	9330
Pimientos, canned, solids and liquid	2300
Pumpkin, raw	1600
canned	6400
Spinach, cooked	8100
Squash, winter, cooked	4200
acorn, baked	1400
butternut, baked	6400
Sweet potatoes, baked in skin	8100
Swordfish, raw	1500
Tomatoes, raw	900
Turnip greens, cooked	6300

29

VITAMIN E

Perhaps no other vitamin has been subjected to such intensive scientific investigation in recent years as vitamin E. All of the investigating efforts have resembled a herd of elephants charging after a mouse, and the results have been about as productive. A lot has been learned about the application of vitamin E to animals and its lack of importance in man. Despite widespread, starry-eyed enthusiasm about vitamin E, its benefits have proved to be more a pious hope than a reality. It has had all of the usual features of a "miracle medicine." And, typically, it has done a great deal more to enrich the pocketbooks of its proponents than to improve the health of the true believers.

Vitamin E was discovered because of its role in improving fertility in rats. I hasten to add that there is no sound scientific evidence that it improves fertility in man, much less either the male's or the female's sexual performance or enjoyment. Of course, it can have the placebo effect enjoyed by any other substance that the true believer has faith in. In experiments, rat fertility improved after vegetable oils and alfalfa and other substances were added to their diet. From this observation vitamin E was discovered and it was given the name of tocopherol. The word comes from the Greek *tokos* meaning childbirth, *pherein* meaning to bear, and the ending *ol* signifying it belongs to the chemical group of alcohol compounds.

Regardless of what vitamin E does for the fertility of rats, it hasn't been proved to do much for man. In fact, medical problems caused by a simple deficiency in vitamin E have yet to be described in either healthy children or adults. Rather, a deficiency occurs as a rare problem in premature infants and apparently in some patients with moderately severe difficulties in absorbing anything from their digestive tract.

The lack of evidence of vitamin-E deficiency, despite the variable diets of human beings, demonstrates how widespread the vitamin is in all of our common foods. This is only part of the picture. Apparently, even if vitamin E is essential for the metabolic processing system, it can be replaced either partially or entirely by other substances, in particular the mineral selenium and the amino acids methionine and cystine. In most of the industrialized nations, where a normal diet would contain adequate quantities of methionine and cystine, it is apparent that the need for vitamin E might not be very great, if it exists at all.

What does vitamin E do? No one yet has definitely proved what vitamin E does in the body, but there are several theories. It appears to be an antioxidant, meaning it prevents the oxygen from destroying other substances. For example, oxygen will cause fats to become rancid; because it prevents this kind of change from oxygen, vitamin E is thought to have some preservative effect. In fact, it can be used as a food preservative in certain circumstances. It is this effect that has led some individuals to claim that vitamin E might have a role in preventing aging. This is a very big might, and no one has proved it, or any unique advantage of vitamin E over any other substances in the antioxidant group. Nothing to date suggests that large doses of vitamin E will perform as an antiaging miracle medicine.

It is possible that vitamin E plays a role with the coenzymes NAD and NADP in the respiratory chain system (the hydrogen express). This, too, may have something to do with the antioxidant effect of vitamin E. A more recent concept, proposed by Dr. Robert Olson of St. Louis University, is that vitamin E is involved in some way in the transfer of information from the vital DNA within the cell nucleus to the rest of the cell. This would affect the cell's capacity for replacement and growth or to perform building processes, including forming new proteins. In this sense vitamin E could be thought of as having a role in growth and growth functions just as does vitamin A. The reason we don't see vitamin-E deficiency and the only reason it doesn't cause cell-growth problems, then, is that our diet includes substances that provide either sufficient vitamin E or enough other substances the body can use as substitutes.

Deficiencies of vitamin E vary enormously depending on which species of animal you're talking about or whether you're talking about man. This is further evidence of the marked individuality of the metabolic systems in different species and the problems of transferring animal vitamin research directly to man. Vitamin-E deficiencies have been associated with difficulties in reproduction and abnormalities of the muscles, bone marrow, liver, brain, and even blood formation. The failure in blood formation as a result of vitamin-E deficiency has been demonstrated only in monkeys and pigs and not in other animals. The sheep and the cow have significant damage to the heart if they have longstanding vitamin-E deficiency. The heart involvement noted in these animals, however, does not occur in monkeys. In the presence of vitamin-E deficiencies in monkeys severe enough to cause marked changes in their skeletal muscles, anemia, and failure of blood formation, no heart involvement has yet been demonstrated. For some reason, even though the skeletal muscles are highly susceptible to vitamin-E deficiencies, the heart muscle is not.

It's important to recognize the different requirements for vitamins in different species. We know that man must get vitamin C because he can't manufacture it from carbohydrates as the cow or dog can. There is no point in feeding a cow vitamin C. Her body will manufacture all she needs. The situation is reversed with vitamin E. The cow must have vitamin E, but man usually gets along very well on minimal amounts. Why? Because the metabolic systems of the cow and man are different. Don't make the mistake of thinking because one animal needs a particular vitamin that all animals and man must also have it. If you follow that erroneous idea all grain and hay-fed animals should be getting vitamin C supplements.

What about using vitamin E as a medicine? The two Dr. Shute brothers of Canada advocated, as early as 1947, that the answer to a host of medical problems was merely giving copious amounts of vitamin E. They recommended that in adolescence one should receive 200 units a day, adult women 400 units a day, adult men and menopausal women 600 units a day, and anyone who had heart disease, vascular disease, or a host of other disorders even much more. A quarter of a century has passed since those initial claims. Several popular books have been published by the enthusiastic Shute brothers, but their claims have not been verified by reputable scientific investigations. This is not because these claims have not received adequate attention. Not only have these claims been evaluated by Dr. Robert Olson, professor of biochemistry at St. Louis University School of Medicine, who has impeccable scientific credentials in both the biochemical and medical fields, but they have also been investigated by such outstanding centers as Boston University, Cornell, Duke, and in England at the University of London and University of Manchester. Despite all of these widespread studies, none has found any benefit in using vitamin E for any of the heart and circulatory problems it has been claimed to benefit.

I would add, however, that for the rare Peyronie's disease, in which a cordlike structure forms in the shaft of the penis causing marked curvature and deformity, a number of urologists have claimed benefits from much smaller doses, in the neighborhood of 25 to 30 units three times a day. There is no universal agreement on this observation, however.

How much vitamin E do you need? One would be tempted, in view of this array of facts, to say that you probably don't need any. It has been generally agreed that some vitamin E should be in the diet, but you won't need more than 15 units. For the most part, you can consider that one unit is equivalent to one milligram. The Food and Nutrition Board, National Academy of Sciences–National Research Council reviewed the problem of vitamin E requirements and revised the RDA values in 1973.

Recommended Daily Allowance of Vitamin E

Children	1–3 years	7 I.U.
	4–6 years	9
	7–10 years	10
Males	11–14 years	12
	over 14 years	15
Females	11–14 years	10
	15–18 years	11
	over 18 years	12
	pregnancy	15
	lactation	15

Is there a toxic reaction to vitamin E? The Food and Drug Administration says that even when adult men take 56,000 units a day for as long as five months no toxic effects are observed. Perhaps one reason for this is that good evidence shows that the body absorbs only the amount of vitamin E it needs in the digestive tract, and most of the rest of it is eliminated with the food residue.

Because of the widespread publicity vitamin E has received, the FDA issued the following statement about it in 1971:

> Clinical trials using vitamin E as a therapeutic agent for many conditions have been reported without conclusive evidence as to the efficacy. Some of these are: habitual abortion, sterility, toxemias of pregnancy, lack of libido, aging, muscular dystrophy, muscle weakness, angina pectoris, coronary heart disease, leg cramps, peripheral vascular disease, and vascular disease.
>
> The FDA is sympathetic to all who are affected by these conditions and joins those who wish vitamin E would be effective as claimed. Unfortunately scientific studies done to back up these claims do not fulfill Federal New Drug Regulation (21CFR 130.12) requirements.

What should you do, then, about vitamin E in your diet? The obvious answer is that unless you're one of those rare individuals with a major problem in absorption from your digestive tract, and you're getting anything like a normal diet, you should forget about vitamin E. If your diet contains sufficient methionine and cystine and reasonable amounts of whole cereal, it is most unlikely that you need concern yourself about additional intake of vitamin E or any special choices of food to provide an adequate amount. Some vitamin-E enthusiasts have claimed you need large amounts of vitamin E if your diet is relatively high in polyunsaturated fats. This doesn't matter either, since the large number of foods rich in polyunsaturated fats are the very ones with the most abundant amounts of vitamin E. Anyone on a diet to prevent atherosclerosis (a relatively low-fat diet with approximately a third of the fat from polyunsaturated sources) is already getting an increased amount of vitamin E.

30

VITAMIN K

The German word for coagulation begins with *k* and that's what vitamin K is all about: blood clotting. It's a very complex vitamin made up of the blocks of carbon, hydrogen, oxygen, and nitrogen. It's another of the fat-soluble vitamins. No one worries very much about how much should be in his diet. A large amount of vitamin K is manufactured by the bacteria in the intestine, and we can absorb this directly into our bodies. The absorption requires bile. Vitamin K is present in reasonably large amounts in pork liver, cabbage, cauliflower, and spinach. It's also been made synthetically, and doctors sometimes use it when too much anti-clotting medicine has been used or in certain medical conditions.

The diet becomes important in reference to vitamin K only if it's a very poor one, such as a soft diet or no food at all, at the same time that antibiotic medicines are given to sterilize the bowel. Since the major source of our vitamin K comes from bacterial action in the intestine, this clearly creates a problem. Sometimes newborns are deficient in vitamin K because their intestines haven't yet developed a normal bacterial flow to produce it.

Vitamin K is used by the liver in the manufacture of several blood-clotting substances, including prothrombin. Apart from this, it doesn't seem to have any other important metabolic actions. When the liver is damaged for any reason, its ability to use vitamin K to form blood-clotting factors can be affected. The absorption of vitamin K is also dependent upon bile flow from the liver. You can see why a patient with liver disease may have a tendency to bleed. Any diarrhea-type disorder that affects absorption can also lead to a vitamin-K deficiency and a tendency to bleeding.

31

VITAMIN D

Vitamin D is known as the antirickets vitamin. Peculiar bone formations and some marked deformities are characteristic of rickets. Vitamin D is directly tied to the body's metabolic processing of calcium and phosphorus.

Vitamin D is the one vitamin that man can obtain from sources other than food. Natural chemical substances in the skin can be activated by the ultraviolet rays of the sun to form vitamin D. It is said that we have enough of these chemicals in three square inches of our skin to supply the daily vitamin-D requirements when they are fully activated by the sun's rays. For this reason, vitamin-D deficiency is essentially unknown in areas of bright sunshine. Some naturalists think man's light skin in the colder climates was an adaptation. The theory is that man's skin was dark until he left warm, sunny climates. Dark pigmentation protects the skin from the sun's rays and prevents the formation of vitamin D. Clearly this would not be a useful function in areas where sunlight is at a premium.

It follows that vitamin-D deficiencies were noted in the cities during cloudy months. The problem became even worse with industrialization as pollution blocked some of the sun's rays. At the turn of the century, approximately 90 per cent of the children in northern-European cities had clinical rickets because of vitamin-D deficiency. The elimination of rickets and other widespread problems through modern food processing has been a major health benefit to modern civilization.

Vitamin D is another complex chemical compound made of carbon, hydrogen, and oxygen. It is put together a lot like cholesterol, and its formation resembles the steroid or sex hormones derived from cholesterol. Two types—vitamin D_2 and vitamin D_3—are important to man, and there is no important distinction between them as far as we're concerned.

Vitamin D is found in liver extract, and in past generations many school children could attest to this from their daily dose of cod-liver oil. It can also be made from a substance called ergosterol found in plants. Ergosterol can be obtained from irradiated yeast, and is a particularly potent source of vitamin D. Vitamin D has been made synthetically. Even if a person must take vitamin D for some reason, it's no longer necessary to take the disagreeable cod-liver oil. And synthetic production of vitamin D has made it possible to enrich many of our foods with it, thus ensuring an adequate intake of vitamin D even for those who live in the less sunny climates. Most milk and milk products today are enriched with vitamin D.

One of the main functions of vitamin D is to increase the intestinal absorption of calcium and phosphorus, necessary for bone formation. Incidentally, the adrenal-cortex hormones tend to antagonize this effect and in this way interfere with growing or maintaining normal bone. By increasing the absorption of calcium and phosphorus through the intestinal wall, vitamin D increases the calcium in the blood. If there is not sufficient vitamin D, the absorption of calcium decreases, and so does the blood calcium. As a result, the four small hormone glands located at the sides of the thyroid, called the parathyroid glands, release a hormone to mobilize calcium from our bones. This brings the blood level of calcium back to normal, but damages the bones. Nature plays some strange tricks on us, and large amounts of vitamin D also tend to cause the calcium to be mobilized from the bones and raises the concentration of calcium in the blood. It's important to maintain an adequate concentration of calcium in the blood and body fluids because calcium is vital to normal cell function. We'll go into that when we discuss the metabolic actions of calcium and other minerals.

For the most part, cereals serve useful functions in the body. They have their ugly side too—cereals, especially oatmeal, aggravate rickets by binding calcium in the intestine so it can't be absorbed. Bile is as essential for the absorption of vitamin D as it is for the other fat-soluble vitamins. It is generally assumed that about half the vitamin D consumed by mouth is eliminated through the food residue.

Vitamin-D deficiencies prevent adequate development of bone, causing rickets. They can also predispose to tooth decay. Under these circumstances, providing sufficient amounts will abolish the problem. In toxic doses, vitamin D mobilizes excess amounts of calcium from the bones and increases the calcium in the blood, causing the formation of calcium deposits in soft tissues where it doesn't belong. This includes collections of calcium in the kidneys and the formation of kidney stones.

How much vitamin D do you need? It is measured in international units, and the RDA for all ages is 400 units. In the United States, because milk and other products are enriched with vitamin D, this quantity is easily obtained from an adequate diet. The margin between having enough and not having enough is relatively narrow for vitamin D, unlike some of the other vitamins. Anyone who is getting four to five times the RDA level is pushing the upper limits of safety. Needs for vitamin D also vary with the amount of sunlight you get. It's not possible, however, to get vitamin D toxicity from sunlight exposure as long as the RDA levels are not greatly exceeded. Most of the problems of vitamin D toxicity occur from excess vitamin-popping, or sometimes in mistakes in mixing prepared foods. The latter problem sometimes occurs in preparing commercial animal food but seldom in human food.

32

IT TAKES CALCIUM
AND PHOSPHORUS TOO

What does the calcium in your body mean to you? Good teeth and strong bones? It does have a lot to do with these, but the bones are only a storehouse for calcium. Active calcium is located in all of our tissues and it's essential to life processes. You need it for normal blood clotting. It affects the electrical activity of the innumerable nerve fibers. It even affects muscle contraction, including the heart muscle. These functions of calcium are so vital that our bones will be robbed of calcium if necessary to keep the calcium level high enough in the blood and body fluids.

Calcium is also important for growth, as you might expect because of its relationship to the skeleton. In classic experiments with twin male rats, one fed a diet containing adequate calcium developed normally. The other rat, on a similar diet but deficient in calcium, was much smaller.

The concentration of the calcium in the blood is the critical factor in controlling the active calcium throughout our body cells. If you eat properly and have a normal body mechanism, you should absorb enough calcium to maintain the blood concentration at the proper level. If you don't, you start losing calcium from your bones. In a healthy adult with adequate stores of calcium, the calcium in the diet should equal the amount lost. We have a tendency to lose some calcium every day, and this must be made up in our dietary intake. The scheme works as in Figure 38.

If your diet includes 1,000 milligrams of calcium, it will be passed into the intestine. About 700 milligrams will be absorbed through the intestinal wall into the bloodstream. This diffuses out into the body fluids to provide the calcium for the metabolic pool for the body. This is not a one-way street. Six hundred milligrams of calcium from the metabolic pool is passed through the intestinal wall back into the intestine. The 600 milligrams that filter through the intestinal wall back inside the intestine mix

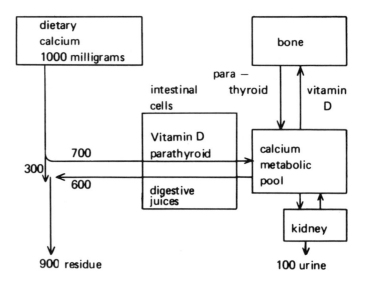

Fig. 38. The calcium balance system.

with the 300 milligrams left over from the calcium in your diet. You now have a balance of 900 milligrams of calcium inside the intestine, and all of this is lost with the food residue. This means that, although you absorbed 700 milligrams of calcium, your net gain was only 100 milligrams. Now if you don't need that 100 milligrams, it would increase the blood calcium too greatly. So it is filtered out through the kidneys into the urine. The end result is that of the 700 milligrams of calcium absorbed, 700 milligrams are eliminated through the bowel and kidneys.

Despite all this action of calcium moving back and forth across the intestine, through the metabolic pool, and being filtered by the kidney, you end up exactly where you started. You will lose calcium through the intestine anyway, and unless you replace it in your diet, you lose more calcium than you take in. When that happens, the bones are robbed of calcium.

There is a constant migration of the calcium in our bones into and out of the blood and body fluids. If your bones are strong, and they stay that way, the amount of calcium that goes in will equal the amount going out. An astonishing one-fifth of the calcium in our bones is turned over every day. Calcium is not taken to the bones and laid down there to stay like a piece of rock, but remains in a constant state of turnover. This explains how you can lose bone so rapidly from the areas around your teeth or from any portion of the skeleton.

Using this little scheme of the traffic pattern for calcium, you can look at the things that affect it. The absorption of that 700 milligrams of calcium through the intestinal wall is achieved through the action of vitamin D and a hormone from the parathyroid gland. These two agents act together to make it possible for us to absorb calcium. If you didn't have any vitamin D or parathyroid hormone, there wouldn't be very much calcium absorbed through the intestinal wall. As a result, you would be losing a lot of calcium from the intestines without replacing it. In short, it would be all outgo and no input.

The exchange between the metabolic pool and the bone calcium bank is also influenced by vitamin D and parathyroid hormone. Vitamin D facilitates the deposit of calcium in the bones in normal circumstances. Parathyroid hormone mobilizes calcium from the bones. In this case, the two are antagonists, and as long as their actions produce equal results the calcium balance deposited in the bone will stay about the same.

Now you can see what happens when you have a vitamin-D deficiency. Not enough calcium will be absorbed, even if your diet is adequate in calcium, and the calcium concentration in the blood and metabolic pool will decrease. This is a critical value and it must be maintained at all costs. If there is insufficient vitamin D to facilitate the deposit of calcium in the bone, the parathyroid hormone helps mobilize calcium out of your bones and adds it to the metabolic pool. This raises the concentration of calcium in the blood. As you see, it's not really very complicated.

The amount of calcium lost in the urine will depend on the amount in the blood. If the calcium level is low, the kidney just stops filtering out calcium. This helps to maintain the blood calcium level.

You can also see what happens when your diet is deficient in calcium. The blood level will fall and the parathyroid hormone will start mobilizing calcium out of the bones to keep it at a safe level for the vital body functions. As a result, your bones will rapidly become decalcified. Any factor that interferes with the absorption of calcium from the intestine will produce the same effect as a low-calcium diet. This includes all the problems of absorption from the intestine. Individuals who have recurrent diarrhea and problems of absorption tend to lose calcium, which in the long run affects the skeleton.

How much calcium do you need? This varies a lot, and certainly if your bones' calcium stores are depleted you'll need more for a while than would usually be required.

Recommended Daily Allowance of Calcium

Children	1–10 years	800 milligrams
Males	11–18 years	1200
	over 18 years	800
Females	11–18 years	1200
	over 18	800
	pregnancy	1200
	lactation	1200

One problem to consider as you get older is dissolving bones. The problem is called osteoporosis (porous bones). It affects the spine and causes that humpbacked appearance so common in women past middle age. About one-fourth of American white women develop this finding. The problem is far more complex than just the amount of calcium in your diet, but it is five times as common in women on a calcium-deficient diet. A high-calcium diet seems to help. Some adults can adjust to a calcium intake as low as 500 milligrams a day. It is risky to assume you are one of them. Osteoporosis is so common in our society that I usually recommend that all teenagers and adults should have 1500 milligrams of calcium in their diet each day. This is the amount of calcium in a quart of fortified skim milk and a little more than in a quart of plain milk.

Your teeth may be the first indication that you need more calcium. Those bad gums associated with absorption of the bone around the teeth (periodontal disease) may be caused by a calcium deficiency. Dr. Lennart Krook and Dr. Leo Lutwak at Cornell have experimental evidence that the first sign of osteoporosis may be those bad gums and loose teeth. I would add here that this isn't the only way this problem can be produced. The Cornell University team says the bone softens around the teeth, then the loose teeth constantly move, damaging the gums. The bone softening was demonstrated by x-rays. By increasing the calcium in the diet, the bone loss was replaced, and the teeth recovered.

The Cornell scientists think the RDA values for calcium for adults are too low—and most people don't get that much calcium in their diet anyway. They have recommended at least 1100 milligrams of calcium for adults. They also think the amount of phosphorus in our diet contributes to the problem. Too much phosphorus limits the use of calcium.

Don't overlook prepared baby-food cereals as a source of calcium. These are particularly useful for older people who already have teeth problems and don't like or won't eat foods normally rich in calcium.

Calcium in Some Common Foods, per 100 Grams (3½ Ounces)

Whole milk, 1 quart	1150	milligrams
Skim milk, 1 quart	1200	
Fortified 2 per cent fat milk, 1 quart	1500	
Fortified skim milk, 1 quart	over 1500	
Nonfat dry milk powder, instant, 1⅓ cups (to make one quart of liquid)	1200	
Milk, canned evaporated, unsweetened, 1 cup	624	
canned condensed, sweetened, 1 cup	801	
Buttermilk, 1 cup	296	
Cheese, natural, blue or Roquefort (3 ounces; 87 grams)	267	
cheddar (1½ ounces; 35 grams)	319	
cottage, creamed, curd pressed down, 1¼ cups (10¾ ounces; 300 grams)	287	
uncreamed, curd pressed down, 1½ cups (10½ ounces; 300 grams)	270	
Parmesan, grated (¾ ounce; 21 grams)	288	
Swiss (1 ounce; 28 grams)	262	
Pasteurized, American (1½ ounces; 43 grams)	297	
Yogurt, 1 cup (8½ ounces; 245 grams)	294	
Bread, white enriched, or whole wheat 1 slice equals 1 ounce	38	
Collards, 3½ ounces (100 grams)	250	
Sardines, 3½ ounces (100 grams) Atlantic (solid and liquids)	354	
Grain solids	437	
Pacific, in tomato sauce (solid and liquids)	449	
Salmon, 3½ ounces (100 grams) canned (solid and liquids) Chum	249	
Coho (silver)	244	
Pink	196	
Red (sockeye)	259	
Beans, 3½ ounces (100 grams) white, mature seeds, cooked	50	
Green peas, 3½ ounces (100 grams) cooked	23	
Soybeans, 3½ ounces (100 grams) immature seeds, cooked	60	
mature seeds, raw	226	

Finally, if you happen to use hard water you may be getting 200 milligrams of calcium a day that way.

Phosphorus is as important as calcium in bone formation. It's present in the bloodstream as phosphate. As you know from the preceding discussions, phosphate is important in the body's metabolism. A large amount of phosphate is essential in the energy scheme within our cells. It is used to form ATP, ADP, AMP, and CP, the basis of our energy system. No wonder the principal salt inside the cell is potassium phosphate.

The concentration of calcium and phosphate in the bloodstream and metabolic pool has a fairly constant value. If the calcium level falls, the phosphate level must rise. When the calcium level rises, the phosphate level falls. In this way, the concentration and its relationship to bones is affected indirectly by vitamin D.

About 20 to 40 per cent of the phosphate in your diet is lost in food residue. Like calcium, the amount of phosphate that is filtered out in the urine depends on the amount of phosphate in the bloodstream. If the concentration in the bloodstream rises, more is filtered out through the kidneys, and if it falls, it's conserved. Parathyroid hormone stimulates the kidney to pour out phosphate.

How much phosphorus do you need in your diet? The RDA values for phosphorus are identical to those for calcium after the first year of life. Usually if you're getting enough calcium in your diet, you will be getting enough phosphorus. Milk is a rich source of both calcium and phosphorus. Many foods have more phosphorus than calcium. A good example is the mature bean seed group. Even the meats are fairly good sources of phosphorus (but poor sources for calcium) because of all that potassium phosphate inside the cells. Our tendency to eat a lot of meat contributes to an excess of phosphorus in the diet compared to our calcium intake. We always think of sweets as a cause of our dental problems. It may be that our meat-eating habits (including chicken and fish) contribute to an unfavorable calcium-phosphorus ratio that causes some of the problems of the soft bones I mentioned. No doubt our ancestors helped solve this problem by chewing on the bone. Milk and milk products have a favorable ratio of calcium to phosphorus, with a little more calcium than phosphorus.

33

THE TRUTH ABOUT MAGNESIUM

Have you ever noticed whenever there's a vacuum in our knowledge about a substance there's a great wave of enthusiasm about its magical qualities? Magnesium certainly fits this description. It is simply a light-weight metallic element and our body certainly requires it. Its exact role in the body hasn't been defined, much less any deficiency state or other health implications affecting the population at large. Magnesium is present in almost all the cells of the body. It seems to be essential to the vital enzyme systems necessary to our metabolic machinery. Within the cell, the magnesium is in the mitochondrion, the area where the glucose, amino acids, fatty acids, and other food items are processed to release their energy.

Magnesium deficiency does occur. It is seen clinically most often in two situations, in the alcoholic and in those who are taking water pills or shots to flush out salt and water. Beyond such abnormal circumstances, the likelihood of a magnesium deficiency seems to be rather remote. This may be because the body is able to stabilize and maintain its magnesium level fairly easily. You have seen that the body is able to maintain a calcium balance. We eliminate the calcium we don't need and conserve or retain calcium when we need it. This general mechanism is character-istic of biological systems unless we purposely do something to upset it. There is no reason to think the situation is any different for magnesium.

There is still some confusion about the absorption of magnesium. Some research studies suggest that calcium tends to block the absorption of magnesium and others suggest that it helps. At this writing, this point has not been clarified.

There are many wild statements about the supposed health benefits of increasing magnesium in the diet. Adelle Davis for one was fond of saying that food raised by organic means is apt to contain more magnesium, which improves health. Research studies on growing plants in various soils show that by using these "organic" methods the magnesium content is actually decreased. She and one or two other prominent individuals who commonly promote large intakes of vitamins and minerals for supposed health benefits have also claimed that magnesium intake lowers blood cholesterol. This claim is not supported by any authentic research studies carried out by reputable scientists. Among the physician-scientist community of heart specialists, there is no support for this concept. It is true that magnesium is important in the function of the heart muscle, and indeed other muscles, but that observation does not mean that the national heart-disease problem is caused by magnesium deficiencies. Not a single expert on heart disease finds any basis for such statements.

There is still some question how much magnesium we do need because we don't know very much about its absorption and elimination from the body, but we do know that it is important in the diet.

Recommended Daily Allowance of Magnesium

Children	1–3 years	150 milligrams
	4–6 years	200
	7–10 years	250
Males	11–14 years	350
	15–18 years	400
	over 18	350
Females	over 10	300
	pregnancy	450
	lactation	450

Magnesium is present, at least in small amounts, in an infinite variety of our foods. This in itself is a probable explanation why clinical magnesium deficiencies are not noted in normal people, even in diets judged to be inadequate for other reasons.

Magnesium in Some Common Foods, per 100 Grams (3½ Ounces)

Mature bean seeds, dry	160 to 180 milligrams
Beef, raw	17 to 22
Most nuts	approx. 200
Cheddar cheese	45
Flounder	30
Lobster	22
Macaroni, cooked	20
Milk	14
Molasses, cane	
light	46
medium	81
blackstrap	258

Magnesium in Some Common Foods, per 100 Grams (3½ Ounces) (Cont.)

Potatoes, raw, unpeeled	34
peeled	22
Salmon, canned	30
Salt	119
Shrimp, boiled	51
Soybeans, mature seed	265
Spinach	88
Turkey, roasted	28
Whole-grain wheat	160
Whole-wheat flour	113
All-purpose white flour	25
Wheat bran, crude	490
Wheat germ	336
Wheat, shredded	133

The fact that magnesium is present in the food doesn't always mean it can be adequately extracted. Spinach, for example, contains a reasonable amount of magnesium, but it also contains oxalate, a substance that binds magnesium in the digestive tract, preventing its absorption. The same is true of many nuts, soybean flour, and wheat germ.

So what should you do about magnesium? Taking additional amounts of magnesium is not likely to have any appreciable influence on its concentration in your body. There doesn't seem to be any advantage in taking more magnesium to supplement your normal diet. If you should be an alcoholic or are taking diuretics to flush out salt and water from your body, your doctor can determine whether you really need more. And if he recommends it he might be well advised not to give you Dolomite tablets, championed by Adelle Davis. These contain both calcium and magnesium and there's some question how well magnesium is absorbed in the presence of calcium.

34

WHY YOU NEED
IRON, MANGANESE,
COBALT, AND COPPER

The popular reason for having "tired blood" is an iron deficiency. Many things cause fatigue, so taking large amounts of iron, either in flavorful syrupy liquids or in any other fashion, won't necessarily eliminate fatigue. Nevertheless, an iron deficiency is one cause of fatigue.

Iron helps form colorful pigments inside and outside the body. One of the most important compounds containing an iron pigment is the hemoglobin in the red blood cells. Hemoglobin is a compound made up of blocks of iron and units of the protein globulin. From what you know about proteins you already know that the globulin has to be made up of a number of amino acids.

Unless your red blood cells contain sufficient hemoglobin, their ability to carry oxygen will be diminished. A significant decrease in the amount of hemoglobin within the red blood cells is an iron-deficiency anemia. In an iron-deficiency anemia you can have a nearly normal number of red blood cells, but they are low in hemoglobin. In pernicious anemia the body just isn't forming enough red blood cells. The total number is decreased, even though each red blood cell may contain a normal amount of hemoglobin. Either condition results in decreased capacity of the blood to transport oxygen to the cells. Now that you understand metabolics, you know this means a decrease in the cell's ability to extract energy from the food. This means less energy for you,.or that old tired feeling. We are back to the basic point that the body's energy depends on an adequate food source for energy, plus an adequate system to process it, which includes adequate amounts of oxygen.

Iron has many other important roles in the metabolic system besides its well-known relation to hemoglobin. It's also part of another compound called myoglobin. This too is made up of iron and globin, but it is a smaller unit than hemoglobin. *Myo* means muscle and this compound is found in our muscles. It combines with oxygen so free oxygen can be available in the muscle cells when we need it. When you start exercising a muscle, this oxygen, already stored in the cell, can be released immediately to run the metabolic processing unit. This provides the working muscle cells with oxygen, and therefore energy, immediately.

The essential cytochrome and cytochrome oxidase of the respiratory chain within each cell (the hydrogen express) also contain iron. You need the iron to transfer hydrogen ripped off the food units along the processing line so it can combine with oxygen and form water. This, as you recall, is closely related to recycling our important coenzymes NAD and NADP, the two main hydrogen carriers. It follows then that the basic energy system of the cell that enables us to use oxygen depends on the presence of a small amount of iron in the body.

Iron seems to be necessary to permit the stomach to release intrinsic factor. Remember, intrinsic factor tacks itself on to vitamin B_{12} so it can be absorbed through the intestinal wall. Since B_{12} is an important growth factor intricately related to the vital cell nucleic acid DNA, you can appreciate how important this function is. Iron is also necessary for formation of our surface cells, including skin, fingernails, and the lining of our digestive tract. Iron deficiency can lead to bright, shiny, inflamed tongue and mucous membranes, fissures around the mouth, and thickening of the lining of the esophagus. This latter problem can be accompanied with problems of swallowing. As you can see, you need iron for a lot more than just "tired blood."

Other than blood transfusions, about the only way you can introduce iron into the body is through the digestive tract. And only about one-tenth of the iron in the diet is ever absorbed through the intestine into the bloodstream. We don't absorb much iron, but under normal circumstances we don't lose much either. The absorption of iron is a very complicated process. A relatively acid environment increases its absorption. Adequate amounts of hydrochloric acid formed by the stomach are important. In older people hydrochloric-acid secretion is decreased and often almost absent. This can lead to difficulties in absorbing iron, causing iron-deficiency anemia. Vitamin C increases iron absorption.

When the body needs more iron it seems to be able to increase the rate of its absorption from food, if everything else is normal. The rest of your diet also influences iron absorption. A relatively low-phosphate diet increases iron absorption, and a high-phosphate diet decreases absorption.

There are differences in the absorbability of various iron preparations. Iron phosphates are absorbed poorly, if at all. And there are two kinds of iron, depending on the complex electrical characteristics of iron itself. One of these is ferrous, the other is ferric. The ferrous preparations are, for example ferrous sulfate, more easily absorbed from the intestine.

Once iron is absorbed into the body, it is stored. Our adult bodies normally contain from 4 to 5 grams of iron, which really isn't very much. Most of this is stored in the liver. This is why liver is a good food source for iron. Large amounts of iron are also found in the intestinal mucous membranes and lesser amounts in the kidney, spleen, and bone marrow.

How much iron do you need in your diet to maintain your metabolic processing system? This depends on how much iron you lose and how much you can absorb from your food sources. Iron requirements vary, but as a guide, mature men require 0.5 to 1.5 milligrams a day. Since only about 10 per cent of the iron in the diet is absorbed, this means most men need from 5 to 15 milligrams a day. The same figure applies to women past menopause. Because of blood loss with menstruation, menstruating women need to absorb 1 to 2.5 milligrams of iron a day to maintain their iron stores. This translates into 10 to 25 milligrams of iron in the diet. The need for iron increases during pregnancy. Not only will the developing baby need iron, but there will be blood loss from the placenta as a result of the delivery. Averaged out on a daily basis, the requirement for iron during pregnancy is between 1.5 and 3.5 milligrams a day, or 15 to 35 milligrams of iron a day in the diet.

Children also need a fairly large amount of iron to build up their iron stores as their body grows. Generally speaking, they need from 1.0 to 1.3 milligrams of iron a day. This means 10 to 13 milligrams a day in their diet. All the recommendations for iron intake should be considered as average.recommendations.

Recommended Daily Allowance of Iron

Infants	6 months	10 milligrams
	6–12 months	15
Children	1–3 years	15
	4–10 years	10
Males	11–18 years	18
	over 18	10
Females	11–50 years	18
	over 50 years	10
	pregnancy	18
	lactation	18

Because of differences in absorbability, and other reasons for losing iron, these values are not always applicable. Furthermore, some women lose more blood during menstruation than others. In these instances, the RDA values may not be sufficient. It's interesting to note the average North American diet contains 12 to 15 milligrams of iron a day.

Another common source of loss of blood is the digestive tract, for example from hemorrhoids. Even losing small amounts of blood every day will have an accumulative effect and increase the iron requirements. Small amounts of blood can be lost from the lining of the colon in individuals who have digestive disturbances. The blood can be mixed with the food residue and, in very small amounts, be relatively unnoticed.

Considering all the variables related to iron absorption and loss, the best way to determine whether a person is getting enough iron is by simple blood tests. The blood hemoglobin test is a good start. If the hemoglobin value is normal, the intake, loss, and storage of iron must likewise be reasonably normal. An exception to this is the person who is on a grossly protein-deficient diet. We need adequate amounts of pro-

Iron in Some Common Foods

Beans, mature seeds, cooked, 1 cup	5.0 milligrams
Green peas, cooked, 1 cup	2.9
Spinach, cooked, 1 cup	4.0
Bread, enriched white or whole wheat 1 slice = 1 ounce	0.7*
Wheat flakes with added nutrients, 1 cup (1 ounce)	1.3
Wheat flour, all-purpose enriched, 1 cup	3.3*
Oatmeal, cooked, 1 cup	1.4
Fish, raw, 3½ ounces (100 grams)	1.0
Sardines, canned, 3½ ounces (100 grams)	10.7
Shrimp, oysters, clams, 3½ ounces (100 grams)	5 to 8
Meat, separable lean, 3½ ounces (100 grams)	3.2
Spleen, hog, 3½ ounces (100 grams)	29.4
beef or calf, 3½ ounces (100 grams)	10.6
Liver, hog, 3½ ounces (100 grams)	19.2
beef, lamb, chicken, 3½ ounces (100 grams)	7 to 10

* Current values. Hearings were begun April 1, 1974, on the proposal to increase these values to 40 milligrams of iron per pound (8.75 milligrams in 100 grams) of enriched flour and 25 milligrams of iron per pound (5.5 milligrams in 100 grams) of enriched bread.

tein to form globin. If for any reason the formation of globin is inadequate, even sufficient iron stores won't result in the formation of enough
hemoglobin. It takes two to tango, iron and globin. So adequate protein
also has a relationship to anemia.

Food preparation also has a lot to do with how much iron we get in
our body. A major and necessary source of iron in the past was all those
iron pots. These are less popular now that enameled-iron, stainless steel,
and aluminum cookware is available. The disappearance of the plain old
iron pot and skillet may decrease the work in the kitchen, but it is far
from an advancement in human nutrition. Even a little rust in the pot
didn't hurt.

Manganese, cobalt, and copper are trace elements that appear to be of
some importance in our metabolic system. Traces of copper serve as a
catalyst in the formation of hemoglobin and appear to have the most
direct application in man. Manganese seems to serve a similar or a
supplemental effect. Cobalt is important in sheep, cattle, and other rumi-
nants because they need it to manufacture vitamin B_{12}. A cobalt deficiency in animals will result in anemia because of vitamin-B_{12} deficiency.

35

IODINE AND YOUR THYROID

An adequate iodine intake is vital to the thyroid gland's main function of forming thyroid hormones, technically known as thyroxine and triiodo-thyronine. The thyroid hormones are formed from iodine and the amino acid tyrosine.

In normal amounts, thyroid hormones stimulate our cells to form protein. Our cells have an assembly system called the microsomes where the amino acids are hooked together to form new proteins for hormones, enzymes, and growth or replacement. Thyroid hormone stimulates these building activities. It works with growth hormone from the pituitary gland to achieve normal growth. In the absence of sufficient thyroid hormone, growth failure occurs. In lower animals it's even important for metamorphosis. A tadpole will not change into a frog unless it has enough thyroid hormone.

Thyroid hormone is also essential to the conversion of beta carotene to vitamin A. It follows that thyroid deficiencies can result in vitamin-A deficiency if the major source for vitamin A is derived from beta carotene found in carrots and pigmented vegetables.

The important coenzyme systems responsible for transporting hydrogen, including NAD, are sensitive to the presence of thyroid hormone. Increased amounts of thyroid hormone cause the hydrogen-carrying NAD to release its hydrogen to oxygen to form water in the normal manner. But an increased amount of energy released in this process is used to form heat, rather than in the formation of energy stored in ATP.

Still another important function of thyroid hormone is its relation to the absorption of carbohydrates from the intestine. Ordinarily, increasing the concentration of glucose in the duodenum will not increase its rate of absorption beyond a relatively low level of concentration. Thyroid hormone increases the ability of the intestinal wall to absorb glucose, and increased amounts of thyroid hormone can cause the blood-glucose level to rise sharply.

Unless a person is taking some medicines that contain iodine, the major source of iodine is the diet. We need a small amount indeed, averaging only about 150 micrograms, hardly more than a trace. It is readily absorbed through the intestinal wall, but once it gets into the circulation it joins the iodine pool. About two-thirds of the amount ingested, or an equivalent amount of iodine in the pool, is eliminated in the urine. The net result is that only about a third of the iodine in the diet is actually retained in the iodine pool so it can be used in the formation of thyroid hormone. You may want to follow the iodine flow diagram (Figure 39).

The blood iodine is carried to the thyroid gland by the circulation, and

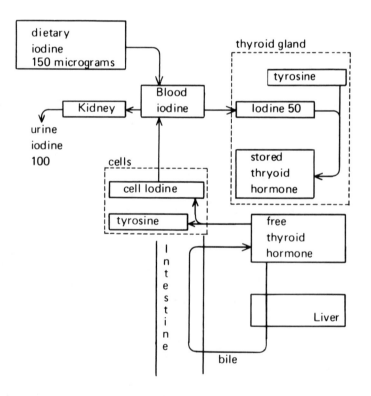

Fig. 39. The iodine balance system.

here it is trapped. Our thyroid gland is made up in lobules. Inside each lobule is a gelatinous colloid material made of protein and carbohydrate (mucoprotein). Accumulations of increased amounts of this produce a colloid goiter. This material is capable of trapping the iodine. Within the thyroid gland, through a number of intricate steps, the iodine is combined with the amino acid tyrosine to form the thyroid hormones. These hormones are released in small amounts into the circulation.

The thyroid gland can store several weeks' supply of thyroid hormone. Once the thyroid hormone is released into the circulation, part of it circulates to the liver where it is processed and passed out of the liver with the bile into the intestine. Some of this is reabsorbed and continues to circulate over and over through the liver. Part of the thyroid hormone in the bile is eliminated with the food residue.

The circulation also carries thyroid hormone to all the cells. In the process of carrying out cell functions, it breaks down into iodine and tyrosine. When the concentration of iodine within the cell is sufficiently high, it is released into the circulation and joins the rest of the iodine pool. From here it can go back to the thyroid for recirculation, or it can join the portion which is eliminated through the urine.

There are only a few sources of iodine in our diet. The principal ones are iodized salt and seafood. Sea water is not a good source of iodine because iodine is present in such minute amounts. However, it is more concentrated in seafood, which provides an excellent source.

If an individual does not have sufficient iodine in his diet, disturbances in thyroid function can occur. This is particularly apt to occur in people who live inland and do not have an iodized-salt source. It was common in the central United States a few decades ago. It has recently been a common problem in Austria and remote mountainous regions that provide their own salt, which is deficient or totally lacking in iodine, and where seafood is not a significant component of the diet. These individuals tend to develop huge goiters. The days when iodine deficiencies were common in the United States preceded my interest in medicine. I was startled when I made a trip to Wagrein, Austria, in 1955 and observed that a large number of the inhabitants of the tiny village had huge thyroid goiters. I was not prepared to see this type of problem, in view of the relatively thorough knowledge about iodine that had existed for several decades.

There are many features of low thyroid function. In its most severe form it can produce coma and death. In general, it is associated with a marked slowing in the body processes. Less food is converted to energy, and the body's need for oxygen is sharply decreased. Oxygen use is commonly measured with the basal metabolic rate test. By demonstrating the low consumption of oxygen, it clearly shows that the metabolic system is not functioning at a normal level. The complete slowing of the body processes results in skin changes, anemia, constipation, mental slowness, changes of the voice, and many chemistry changes.

There is a gradual decrease in the output of thyroid hormone with increasing years, and this may be one factor related to obesity with middle age. However, low thyroid function is rarely a significant factor in obesity today. The indiscriminate administration of thyroid medicine in the treatment of obesity has no sound physiological basis. If thyroid hormone is administered in small amounts to a person who has a normal thyroid gland, the gland just quits putting out as much hormone as it used to. The smaller amount put out by the normal thyroid gland plus that taken by mouth equals the amount that would have been produced if the situation had been left alone. Because the thyroid gland cuts back on its production, once the hormone is discontinued there will be a period of sluggishness and fatigue. It takes several weeks for the thyroid to resume its normal level of function. This development of symptoms when thyroid hormone is stopped often leads individuals to be erroneously convinced that the thyroid hormone was essential.

When an excess amount of thyroid hormone is formed, the opposite effects occur. Metabolism is greatly stimulated, and the process involving the hydrogen carrier NAD results in the release of energy as heat rather than in the formation of ATP. Because the process is accelerated, individuals with overactive thyroids feel hot, but their energy level may actually be decreased. These persons have developed an inefficient machine which is overheating. The energy is no longer being used for power for the multiple needs of the body, such as the formation of protein. It's much as if your electric light bulb quit putting out light from its electrical energy and used the current solely for heat production.

Under these circumstances, there is a rapid turnover of energy materials in the body. People with an overactive thyroid eat large amounts of food, but a lot of the calorie value of the food is wasted as heat. There will be no significant weight gain, despite the enormous amount of calories consumed. If the calorie intake can't meet the stepped-up rate, the body starts digesting itself. Proteins are mobilized from the muscles and utilized, and the fat stores in the body are depleted. Associated with these changes, the excess thyroid hormone mobilizes calcium from the bone and increases the loss of calcium and phosphorus in the urine. It's not surprising under these altered metabolic circumstances that muscles and nerves become hypersensitive. There may be muscle spasms and an overactive nervous system even associated with emotional instability. Of course, these stepped-up metabolic activities in the cell require an adequate supply of oxygen. This means the circulation has to step up its work to provide more oxygen to the cells, accounting for the increased heart rate common in these problems.

36

YOU NEED SALT AND WATER

The amount of salt and water in your body is of vital importance to how you feel. A loss of sodium from the body can cause you to feel exceptionally fatigued. Too much sodium salt can cause the body to retain excess water, causing swelling in the tissues, and is one of many causes for swollen ankles. Accumulation of fluid in the lungs can affect breathing. The various salts and water have a great deal to do with how acid your body is. The body's chemical processes depend on maintaining the balance between acid and alkaline substances within a very narrow range. Our body is neither acid nor alkaline, but very nearly neutral.

The important salts in the body water outside the cells, including the blood, are chloride salts. These include ordinary sodium chloride (simple table salt), potassium chloride (sometimes used as a salt substitute with another element added to give it a better taste), and much smaller amounts of calcium and magnesium salts. The other large group of salts outside the cell are bicarbonates. The classic example here is ordinary sodium bicarbonate, familiar to every housewife. Contributing to the overall pool of chemical salts are phosphates, sulfates, and those important organic acids, including the ketone bodies, such as acetoacetic acid.

Sodium and potassium salts are probably the best-known salts. The watery solution in our blood and surrounding all of the body cells contains about the same amount of sodium as ordinary sea water. This is about the same concentration found in most animals.

There is very little sodium chloride inside the cells. The main salt here is potassium phosphate and a small amount of potassium bicarbonate. This is not too surprising, since phosphate sources are constantly needed to interact in the formation of ATP and the energy system.

None of these salts has any caloric value. They separate into individual building blocks of sodium, chloride, potassium, and phosphate, rather han remaining together as a single unit in the solid form familiar to us. The concentration of sodium and potassium has a lot to do with the cells' response to the basic materials calcium, magnesium, and phosphorus. These salts also enter into complex relationships with the metabolic processing system. If the concentration of any of them is too high or too low, difficulties can occur. Even when salts are present in their right concentration, the total volume of fluid has to be correct as well. A person can be dehydrated or overhydrated and still have a normal concentration of salt. The amount of water in the body, under normal circumstances, tends to be controlled by the amount of sodium we retain.

Many factors affect sodium retention. The one most familiar to women is the swelling they experience just preceding the menses. The increased formation of female hormones causes the body to retain sodium. To prevent too high a concentration of sodium, the body then retains water, causing premenstrual swelling. Heart failure, liver disease, and kidney disease are all capable of causing sodium and water retention responsible for swellings.

Normally you can vary your salt intake a great deal, and the kidneys simply eliminate what you don't need. These mechanisms are fairly complex, but the end result is fairly simple. If you use a lot of salt, you will drink a lot of fluids. This dilutes the sodium sufficiently for it to be properly eliminated by the kidneys. You'll simply wash out the excess sodium along with the excess water. Potassium is not directly tied to the retention of body fluid, but excess amounts of it also are eliminated through the kidneys. Water, sodium, potassium, chloride, and the entire group of salts and water tend to be kept in proper balance by the function of the kidneys.

The kidneys' functions aren't the only way of controlling this balance. Large amounts of sodium can be lost during heavy sweating, particularly in a person who is not acclimatized to heat. When the water and salt loss is replaced solely with water, a low sodium concentration state eventually occurs, causing severe fatigue and sometimes muscle cramps. This is not common, as is popularly believed, but does occur in hot climates during heavy labor in individuals who sweat excessively. Severe diarrhea can also cause a loss of salts and water, greatly disturbing the balance and total amount in the body.

You may be surprised to know that much of the initial weight loss from fad diets is related to a sudden loss of sodium. Simple fasting or any diet which involves the excessive elimination of carbohydrates causes the kidneys to lose their ability to retain sodium. Sudden flushing out of the sodium salts carries with it a lot of body water and the dieter is enthusiastic about the results of the new regime. But unfortunately this loss has nothing to do with the stores within the fat cells and is not equated to a loss of stored calories. As soon as a normal dietary pattern is reestablished, adequate sodium will be retained and with it the normal amount of water. Of course, the body weight will return to its previous levels, unless something more meaningful has been accomplished in the way of eliminating calories. During this type of diet potassium loss may also occur.

With severe fasting, diabetic acidosis, and the no-carbohydrate diet recommended by Dr. Atkins for the first week of his program, abnormal amounts of ketone bodies are formed. These acids tend to deplete the body's store of sodium and water. Obviously, another example of how the sodium and potassium can be depleted is by the use of diuretics or water pills. These are commonly used in the treatment of heart failure, sometimes used to eliminate premenstrual accumulations of water, and may be used in the treatment of high blood pressure.

The potassium-sodium concentrations and the total electrolyte picture, including the electrical activity of our cells, are important in normal cell function. Too high a concentration of potassium can cause the heart to stop entirely. Too low a concentration of potassium leads to irregularities of the heart, including some that are serious or even fatal.

Although the total role of the salts and water in regulating the acid-base balance of the body is complex, some of the basic principles are fairly simple. Ordinary baking soda or sodium bicarbonate helps protect the body from being overwhelmed by acid. Let's consider the possibility of adding excess hydrochloric acid, a strong acid, to the body. The sodium bicarbonate and hydrochloric acid simply interact to form sodium chloride and carbonic acid, a weak acid. Remember that carbonic acid is merely a unit of water and a unit of carbon dioxide. If too much carbonic acid is accumulating in the body, it can be broken down to water and carbon dioxide and eliminated through the lungs and kidneys.

A strongly alkaline substance such as sodium hydroxide (one block of sodium, one block of oxygen, and one block of hydrogen) interacts with carbonic acid to form sodium bicarbonate and a unit of water. The carbonic acid and sodium bicarbonate together in our fluids are able to keep the chemical balance from being overwhelmed by either strong acid or strong alkaline substances. As excess amounts of a substance such as sodium chloride are formed, they can be eliminated from the body. Far more complex methods are involved here which include phosphate salts and complex chemistry, but the simple principle expressed above is the end result. In order to preserve the delicate acid-alkaline balance in the body, it's important to have the right amounts of the various salts and water.

There are abundant sources of sodium chloride in our diet. Usually the problem is not how to obtain sufficient amounts, but rather how to avoid getting too much. Unfortunately, many of us love the taste of salt and would consider our food tasteless without it. Even so, a knowledge and expert use of spices in cooking helps enormously in restricting salt intake.

Although there's great variation in how much salt is used by different individuals, the average daily intake of sodium chloride in the United States per person is 10 to 12 grams. This is well in excess of our daily need, which for adults is probably no more than 2.5 grams.

Sodium is present in an abundant amount in almost all animal products. After all, any meat we eat comes from an animal which has the same kind of water in its tissues as we do. Ordinarily milk also contains a large amount of sodium. There is an appreciable amount of sodium in a number of vegetables. On the other hand, fruits are relatively low in sodium and very high in potassium. Salt is usually added in cooking and sometimes again at the table.

You can achieve a major reduction in salt intake by eliminating all salt used in food preparation and being sure not to buy prepared foods that already have salt added. For the benefit of those rare individuals who need to be on a low-sodium diet, the following foods are low in sodium:

Fruits, berries, melons, (raw or canned)
Vegetables (raw or prepared without salt)
Mature bean seeds, soybeans, nuts (raw or prepared without salt)
Flour, all types except self-rising
Cereals (raw or prepared without salt)

The important meat group contains a moderate amount of sodium.

Sodium in Meat (Raw), per 100 Grams (3½ Ounces)

Beef	65 milligrams
Chicken	60
Fish (not shellfish)	70
Lamb	75
Pork (not cured)	70
Turkey	65
Veal	90

Foods Moderately High in Sodium

Milk, whole, 1 cup (8 ounces)	120 milligrams
Cheese, cottage, 3½ ounces (100 grams)	
creamed	229
uncreamed	290
Cheese, cream, 3½ ounces (100 grams)	250
Egg, whole, one	122
Shrimp, 3½ ounces (100 grams)	140
Scallops, 3½ ounces (100 grams)	255

The following foods should be considered high-sodium foods. They should be used sparingly, if at all, when salt restriction is necessary:

Foods High in Sodium

Baby foods, except fruits
Baking powder
Bacon
Barbecue sauce
Beef, corned or dry
Biscuits, breads, rolls, buns, muffins
Breakfast cereals, commercial
Butter, salted
Buttermilk
Cakes
Candies (most)
Cheese, processed
Cocoa and chocolate-beverage powders
Cookies
Cornmeal, self-rising
Crackers, except dietetic
Gelatin, dessert powder
Lobster
Margarine, salted
Mustard
Olives
Peanut butter
Chili powder with added salt
Pickles
Relish
Pies
Pizza
Pork and cured ham
Pudding, pudding mix
Salad dressings
Salmon, canned (unless canned without salt)
Sandwich spread
Sardines
Sauerkraut
Sausages, luncheon meats, cold cuts, frankfurters
Soups
Tartar sauce
Tomato catsup
Tomato chili sauce
Tomato juice
Tuna, canned (unless canned without salt)
Vegetables, canned or commercially prepared or cooked with salt
Waffles
Wheat flour, self-rising

You might want to know that a level teaspoon of table salt contains about 2500 milligrams of salt. Some city water and "softened" water contains significant amounts of sodium. Mature bean seeds and soybeans are particularly important because they are high in protein, even though hey are low in sodium. This combination is hard to come by in food. Roasted soybeans would be one way to increase the protein intake in the diet without appreciably increasing the sodium intake.

The problem with potassium is exactly the opposite. Very often individuals who are taking diuretics will wash out not only sodium, but also too much potassium. Healthy individuals on a normal diet usually will have no problem about potassium. For those individuals with medical problems that result in low potassium, it's important to include in the diet foods high in potassium, and this means fruits.

You might like to know that three glasses of orange juice a day will provide as much potassium as most doctors usually prescribe to replace potassium loss. Individuals taking diuretics or digitalis for heart failure who do not have kidney problems could include in their diet generous amounts of orange juice, or ruby-red grapefruit, as well as other fruits.

37

HOW TO PLAN
A HEALTHY DIET

With the knowledge of what the body does with your food, you should now be able to plan a healthy diet designed to provide you with the maximum amount of energy. All the calories, vitamins, and minerals essential for running our body in its optimal state are available in our food sources. Not everyone takes full advantage of these, most often because of lack of information.

If you plan your diet properly, there should be no need to take additional vitamins, minerals, or other supplements. Just keep in mind, there is no energy in either vitamins or minerals. The individuals who benefit from vitamin and mineral supplements are those who do not have sufficient amounts in their diet. This automatically means their diet is inadequate. I would hope my statement is not construed to mean that vitamin and mineral preparations are not important. They certainly are. In certain situations they are an important adjunct to the diet in maintaining health. In the main, though, these circumstances occur in individuals who are ill or who have poor dietary habits for one reason or another. Certainly anyone who has a vitamin deficiency initially will need increased amounts of vitamins and minerals until the situation has been adequately corrected.

It is rather ironic that some of the well-known individuals who are most vocal about the role of food and health are also vitamin gurus. Often they advocate nutritious foods as a means to health and almost in the next sentence advocate vitamin pills and minerals to "prop up that sagging energy." The obvious contradiction doesn't slow down many of these self-appointed, so-called authorities. If you want to avoid this kind of hoax, you need solid basic information on nutrition and a solid understanding of what your body does with food.

Just remember that when one of the vitamin gurus starts advocating vitamins for you, he or she is assuming your diet is not adequate or that you have an underlying medical problem preventing adequate absorption of vitamins. Unless such a person knows what your medical status is and what your dietary habits are, he or she is not in a position to make such judgments. The same applies to protein supplements. If you plan your diet right, and it's a good one, it ought to contain sufficient amounts of protein with adequate amounts of essential amino acids. If for any reason your diet is not providing adequate amounts of protein, protein supplements are useful.

Let's take a look at the main objectives of a healthy diet plan. You can really put them into five categories.

1. To provide sufficient calories as the source of energy for your body.

2. To provide sufficient protein, adequate in all of the amino acids, to provide the basic building blocks for the body's processes of building tissues, hormones, enzymes, and carrying out essential body functions.

3. To provide a minimum of 50 grams of carbohydrate a day sufficient to enable the body to carry out its chemical processes without causing a chemical imbalance, such as the excess formation of ketones causing acidosis.

4. To provide a minimal amount of fat, which can hardly be avoided anyway, to enable the absorption of the fat-soluble vitamins, principally vitamins D and A. The small amount of fat necessary should include very small amounts of the polyunsaturated fats.

A healthy diet should limit the proportion of fat and cholesterol (which is not a fat, but is classified in the lipid group). Your fat intake should be less than 35 per cent of the total calories ingested. Less than 10 per cent of the total calories should come from saturated fats while approximately 10 per cent of the total calories should be polyunsaturated fat. The cholesterol should not exceed 300 milligrams a day.

5. A sufficient variety of foods should be included in the menu to provide adequate amounts of all the vitamins and minerals. Remember, these substances are used as catalysts for the food energy system or, as in the case of calcium and phosphorus, in bone structure.

With this maze of facts you would be justified in wondering what in the world you can do about planning an adequate diet. Nutritionists have solved this problem by considering all these facts and generalizing our food into four basic groups. The idea is that you should obtain sufficient foods from each of the four basic groups to have a fairly balanced diet. These four basic groups are the dairy products, the meat group, the cereal and bread group, and the fruit and vegetable group. To help you plan your menus and eating habits, let's go through each one of these groups and consider what it contributes to the diet and which ones are best to meet the basic objectives of a healthy diet plan.

The dairy-products group means milk and milk products. They are the major source of calcium in our diet and also provide phosphorus. You can get a large amount of phosphorus from other products, but it's more difficult to obtain the calcium. In addition, the milk products provide an important diet source of complete protein, meaning that the protein will include all the essential amino acids. The butterfat in any of these milk products naturally contains vitamins A and D. In recent years, dairy products have been enriched with A and D to increase the amount of these vitamins in the usual diet of the greatest number of people. Individuals who are accustomed to eating lots of fruits and vegetables will easily meet their requirements for vitamin A without relying on those in milk and milk products. Those who live in very sunny climates will tend to get enough vitamin D just from climatic exposure. However, the addition of vitamin D to milk products helps ensure that individuals in the smog-laden, industrial Northern cities will have regular adequate amounts of vitamin D. Milk also contains thiamine. You can obtain 0.4 milligrams of thiamine from a quart of low-fat or skim milk fortified with 2 per cent nonfat milk solids. Cottage cheese in the amounts listed also provides significant amounts of thiamine. The other cheeses do not. As a general rule for planning your diet, the daily intake for an adult should include four of the following items:

Milk, whole, 3.5 per cent fat, 1 cup (8½ ounces; 244 grams)	160 calories
2 per cent low-fat, 2 per cent nonfat milk solids added, 1 cup (8½ ounces; 246 grams)	145
skim, 1 cup (8½ ounces; 245 grams)	90
skim, 2 per cent nonfat milk solids added 1 cup (8½ ounces; 245 grams)	105
canned, evaporated, unsweetened ½ cup (4½ ounces; 126 grams)	172
condensed, sweetened ⅓ cup (3½ ounces; 100 grams)	327
nonfat, dry powder, ⅓ cup (1 ounce; 29 grams)	82
Milk substitute—ProSobee (Mead Johnson) 1 cup (8 ounces; 240 grams)	160
Buttermilk, from skim milk, 1 cup (8½ ounces; 245 grams)	90

Cheese, natural, blue or Roquefort
   (3 ounces; 87 grams)   315
   cheddar (1½ ounces; 35 grams)   172
   cottage, creamed, curd pressed down,
   1¼ cups (10¾ ounces; 306 grams)   305
   uncreamed, curd pressed down
   1½ cups (10½ ounces; 300 grams)   255
   Parmesan, grated (¾ ounce; 21 grams)   98
   Swiss (1 ounce; 28 grams)   105
   Pasteurized, American (1½ ounces;
   43 grams)   157
   Swiss (1 ounce; 28 grams)   100
Yogurt, 1 cup (8½ ounces; 245 grams)   125

Remember, these items can be included in food preparation, such as gravies, white sauce, mashed potatoes, puddings and baked goods, or breakfast cereals. If you meet this requirement from the milk group, you'll get about 1200 milligrams of calcium. This will exceed the RDA for calcium needs.

Any of the items in the milk group will provide a lot of excellent complete protein. Each glass of milk or buttermilk will contain about 9 grams of protein; creamed cottage cheese, 41 grams; uncreamed cottage cheese, 50 grams; every other cheese item, 8 to 10 grams; and yogurt, 7 to 8 grams of protein. You can't fail to get over 30 grams of complete protein by including any four units of these foods in your diet.

If you need to control the amount of fat in your diet, and most people do, you can use the low-fat items: fortified skim milk, buttermilk, nonfat dry milk powder, and uncreamed cottage cheese. You can also decrease the amount of these items if you have a suitable substitute for calcium, such as sardines or canned salmon eaten with the bones. Uncreamed cottage cheese is a low-fat item, creamed cottage cheese is a moderate-fat item, and the rest of the cheeses are very high-fat foods, with about half the fat saturated fat.

The meat group is a major source of complete protein. Since the amino acids in meat are very close to the percentages and arrangements found in our muscles, they are readily used in an efficient manner. There is almost nothing in the meat group that can't be obtained from other foods, except protein. And you can get adequate protein without meat by using milk products and the bean group. The small amounts of iodine our body requires can be obtained from fish, shellfish, or salt. As you can tell from the discussions of the various vitamins, certain meat items, usually organ meats, are good sources of vitamins. Liver is a good source of iron. Pork is a good source of thiamine. Many of the meats are not particularly good sources for vitamins or minerals, and in this respect are often inferior to vegetables, fruits, and cereals, but they are unbeatable in the protein department. The meat group includes all the mammal meats (beef, pork, and lamb), fish, shellfish, and poultry. In some parts of the world you could add to that the reptile group.

Although there is a slight variation in different cuts of meat, and whether it is chicken, fish, lamb, or turkey, for planning purposes think of this group as being 18 per cent protein (5 grams of protein per ounce of flesh or 18 grams per 100 grams). This also applies to shellfish with the exception of oysters—they have about half as much protein, so double the amount of oysters by weight to provide the same amount of protein. It follows that you want to include two servings of 3½ ounces (100 grams) each in your daily menu of any of these items. The 7 ounces (200 grams) can all be in one meal or divided. Remember this applies only if the daily menu also includes the recommended amount of milk products. If no milk products are used, it would be advisable to increase the meat group in the menu to four servings or a total of 14 ounces (400 grams).

A practical problem is how to determine the weight of flesh in ready-to-cook poultry. As a guide, estimate that a third of the weight will be bones. You can use this figure for either chicken or turkey. If you want a 4-ounce serving of chicken, you should cook 6 ounces. If the ready-to-cook weight of a bird is 3 pounds, the edible part will only be 2 pounds.

Plan your meat group to avoid too much saturated fat and to provide sufficient amounts of polyunsaturated fat. You can do this by rotating the items so that one-third of the group comes from mammal meat, one-third from fish, and one-third from poultry.

Do you want to use meat substitutes? You might, with the world-wide shortage of items in the meat group. The milk group is an obvious meat substitute for protein. Don't forget that many animals are raised on milk as the major protein source during their active growth phase. You can substitute uncreamed cottage cheese, ounce for ounce or gram for gram for the meat group and get the same amount of complete proteins. Creamed cottage cheese doesn't contain quite as much protein and you should use a fourth more (5 ounces of creamed cottage cheese for 4 ounces of meat or 5 grams for 4 grams). It is a cheap substitute in most areas.

The bean group should not be used alone, at least for growing children. But it is all right if you also use the proper amount of the dairy group for complete proteins, or include plenty of cereals in the diet. For planning purposes, estimate that you will need twice as much cooked mature bean seeds as you would need of meat (raw weight). In other words, the cooked weight of the beans should be 200 grams to replace 100 grams of raw meat. In the absence of milk and milk products, the meatless diet should include adequate amounts of cereal in combination with beans.

Eggs contain good protein, but they also contain a lot of cholesterol and usually considerable amounts of saturated fat. Two eggs weigh 3½ ounces (100 grams), and since they are 12 per cent protein you would need three eggs to equal the amount of protein in a serving of the meat group. That would also introduce over 700 milligrams of cholesterol into the diet. You can avoid this problem by using only egg whites, but it takes four to five egg whites to equal the protein in a serving of meat. You can add large numbers of egg whites to almost any baked product, including homemade bread, to increase egg-white consumption. Some people can increase the quality of protein in their diet by using whole eggs. The problem here, basically, is the high concentration of cholesterol in the egg yolk. Also, the percentage of calories from fat in the egg yolk is high. Because of the fat-cholesterol-atherosclerosis problem, before depending on eggs for protein it's a good idea to check with your doctor. You shouldn't use many egg yolks unless your doctor tells you it's all right. Some individuals have low cholesterol levels, and the amount of egg yolk in their diet may not be particularly important. This may be true in young children (but certainly not all; many have high cholesterol levels in early childhood) and in menstruating women.

A doctor should not recommend using large amounts of egg yolks unless he has thoroughly studied the blood fat and cholesterol content and is completely satisfied these values are in the lower level. Specifically, the blood cholesterol level should be 200 or less with no elevation of the triglycerides (fats). Such individuals are not likely candidates for heart and vascular disease. The blood tests should be repeated at frequent intervals to be certain the values haven't changed, making it unwise to continue using lots of eggs.

The third basic food group includes cereals and bread. You should think of this group as the vitamin B, vitamin E, and mineral group. It is also a major source of bulk in the diet, important for digestion and controlling the rate of absorption. There are important amounts of protein and polyunsaturated fats within the bread and cereal group. Because milk products are used in making bread items, they actually provide both cereal and milk products for the diet. Since even breakfast cereals are commonly eaten with milk, they too fall into this category. Some of the prepared cereals have iron added in the enrichment process. To provide a well-balanced diet, the daily menu should include at least one of the items in the amount listed. For growing boys and those with a high thiamine requirement I recommend a minimum of two items, in the quantity listed, each day. The items with the calories for each are:

Biscuits, dinner rolls, muffins, 3	300 calories
Bread, 3 slices (1 slice = 1 ounce; 28 grams)	225
Macaroni, enriched, cooked, 1 cup (5 ounces; 140 grams)	155
Noodles (egg noodles) cooked, 1 cup (5½ ounces; 160 grams)	200
Pancakes, 4-inch diameter, 4 cakes (1 cake = 1 ounce; 28 grams)	240
Spaghetti, enriched, cooked, 1 cup (5 ounces; 140 grams)	155
Waffles, 7-inch diameter, 1½ waffles (2⅔ ounces; 75 grams)	310
Bran flakes (40 per cent bran) with added thiamine and iron, 1½ cups (1¾ ounces; 53 grams)	160
Cornflakes, with added nutrients, 1⅔ cups (1½ ounces; 42 grams)	166
Farina, quick-cooking, enriched, cooked, 1½ cups (13 ounces; 368 grams)	160
Oats, puffed, with added nutrients, 1 cup (less than 1 ounce; 25 grams)	100
Oatmeal, cooked, 1 cup (8½ ounces; 240 grams)	130
Rice, white, enriched, cooked, 1 cup (over 7 ounces; 205 grams)	225
Wheat, puffed, with added nutrients, 2½ cups (1⅓ ounces; 38 grams)	137
Wheat, shredded, plain, 3 biscuits (2⅔ ounces; 75 grams)	270
Wheat flakes, with added nutrients, 1 cup (1 ounce; 30 grams)	105

You can see why a breakfast of cereal is an advantage. It is a way to provide needed items from this list for a balanced diet. Without cereal or bread items for breakfast it may be difficult to provide enough thiamine for the daily needs. While meat contains some thiamine, except for pork products it is not a rich source for it. A cereal breakfast, using fortified skim milk, combined with fresh fruit or fruit juice is an excellent way to start the day. It also provides bulk. The only exception to this is those individuals who have a problem in reactive low blood glucose. These individuals are a special case and require a different approach to menu planning. If they are unable to utilize cereals and breads, they may need to take vitamin supplements.

The fourth important food group includes vegetables, fruits, melons, and berries. This group is rich in vitamins A and C. You might want to check your list of common foods containing vitamin A and C in those chapters. Some of these items also contain significant amounts of the vitamin B group, and they are an important source of minerals. Although it's conceivable that you can satisfy your vitamin A, B, and D requirements from the other three basic food groups, you will have trouble meeting the daily vitamin-C requirements unless your diet contains enough vegetables and fruits.

It is a good idea to subdivide this large group. I divided the vegetables into the legume-nut subgroup, the leafy subgroup, and the miscellaneous subgroup. That leaves the fruit, berry, and melon subgroup.

Each of the items on the legume and nut list contains about 0.2 milligram of thiamine. Green peas and beans are fairly common foods. You should have at least one of the food items on this list each day.

Beans, mature seeds, cooked, drained, 1 cup (5⅓ ounces; 180 grams)	225 calories
Beans, immature lima seeds, cooked, drained, ⅔ cup (4 ounces; 115 grams)	127
Soybeans, immature seeds, boiled, drained, ⅔ cup (3½ ounces; 100 grams)	118
mature seeds, raw or dry-roasted (¾ ounce; 20 grams)	80
Cowpeas, blackeyed peas, lentils, mature seeds, cooked, drained, ½ cup (4½ ounces; 125 grams)	88
Peas, green, cooked, drained, ½ cup (2¾ ounces; 80 grams)	58
Almonds, ⅔ cup (3 ounces; 90 grams)	566
Peanuts, roasted, ½ cup (2½ ounces; 70 grams)	420
Pecans, ¼ cup (1 ounce; 27 grams)	185

Each item in the leafy vegetable subgroup contains only about 0.1 milligram of thiamine. You can get your salads from the lettuce. You should have at least two of the items from this list in your menu each day.

Broccoli, cooked, ⅔ cup (3½ ounces; 100 grams)	27 calories
Brussels sprouts, cooked, ½ cup (5¼ ounces; 155 grams)	55
Cabbage, raw, finely shredded, 2 cups (6¼ ounces; 180 grams)	40
Cauliflower, cooked, 1 cup (4¼ ounces; 120 grams)	25
Collards, cooked, ⅓ cup (2¼ ounces; 65 grams)	28
Dandelion greens, cooked, 1½ cups (3 ounces; 90 grams)	30
Lettuce, crisp head (iceberg) ⅓ head (5¼ ounces; 150 grams)	20
Mustard greens, cooked, 1 cup (less than 5 ounces; 140 grams)	35
Sauerkraut, canned solids, 1½ cups (12¼ ounces; 350 grams)	68
Spinach, cooked, with liquids, 1 cup (6¼ ounces; 180 grams)	40
Turnip greens, cooked, ⅔ cup (3½ ounces; 100 grams)	20

The miscellaneous vegetable group includes a number of important common foods. Each item contains only 0.1 milligram of thiamine, and you should include at least two of these items in your diet each day.

Asparagus, green, cooked, ½ cup (2¾ ounces; 75 grams)	15 calories
Beans, green or wax, cooked, drained, 1 cup (4½ ounces; 125 grams)	30
Corn, sweet, cooked kernels, drained, over 1 cup (3½ ounces; 100 grams)	83
Carrots, diced, cooked, 1 cup (5¼ ounces; 145 grams)	45
Okra, cooked, ½ cup (over 3 ounces; 90 grams)	26
Parsnips, cooked, 1 cup (5¼ ounces; 155 grams)	100
Potatoes, baked or boiled with peel, 1 potato (3½ ounces; 100 grams)	90
French fried (3½ ounces; 100 grams)	290
Pumpkin, canned, 1½ cups (12 ounces; 342 grams)	342
Squash, summer, cooked, 1 cup (over (7 ounces; 210 grams)	30
winter, baked, 1 cup (7 ounces; 205 grams)	130

Sweet potatoes, cooked, before peeling
    (4 ounces; 115 grams)   160 calories
Tomatoes, raw, 1 (7 ounces; 200 grams)   40
    canned, 1 cup (8½ ounces; 240 grams)   50
Tomato juice, 1 cup (8½ ounces;
    240 grams)   45

Each item in the fruit, berry, and melon group contains about 40 milligrams of vitamin C. Use two of these items each day and your diet will exceed the RDA for vitamin C.

Blackberries, raw, 2 cups (10½ ounces;
    300 grams   170 calories
Blueberries, raw, 2 cups (10 ounces;
    280 grams)   170
Cantaloupe, raw, ⅓ melon (9 ounces;
    250 grams)   40
Cranberry juice, 1 cup (9 ounces;
    250 grams)   170
Grapefruit, raw, half of 3¾-inch diameter
    (17 ounces; 480 grams with rind)   44
Grapefruit juice, ½ cup (4⅔ ounces;
    62 grams)   46
Lemon, raw, 1 whole (4 ounces; 110 grams
    with rind)   20
Lemon juice, ½ cup (4¼ ounces;
    122 grams)   30
Orange, raw, ⅔ (4½ ounces; 120 grams
    with peel)   45
Orange juice, ⅓ cup (less than 3 ounces;
    82 grams)   36
Papaya cubes, raw, ½ cup (3¼ ounces;
    90 grams   35
Pineapple, raw, diced, 2 cups (10 ounces;
    280 grams)   150
Pineapple juice, 2 cups (17½ ounces;
    500 grams)   270
Raspberries, raw, 1⅓ cups (5½ ounces;
    164 grams)   105
Strawberries, raw, ½ cup (2¾ ounces;
    7 grams)   28
Tangerine, raw, 1 medium (4¼ ounces;
    120 grams, with peel)   40
Tangerine juice, ½ cup (4½ ounces;
    125 grams)   62
Watermelon (about 2⅔ pounds,
    1.2 kilograms with rind, or 1/12 of a
    10 × 16-inch melon)   150

The lists I have given you provide the basis for planning a healthy diet. By selecting the appropriate number of items from each group, you will meet the objectives of providing sufficient quality protein, carbohydrates, bulk, vitamins, minerals, and polyunsaturated fats.

In the interest of limiting fat intake in the diet, it's important to look at methods of food preparation, avoiding the excess use of fat, such as occurs in deep-fat frying, or the use of fats in salad dressings and vegetable preparation. These hidden fat sources may cause the percentage of calories from fat intake in the diet of industrialized nations to be over 50 per cent of the total number consumed. To have a moderately low-fat, low-cholesterol diet, you should avoid excessive use of nuts. In this group, avoid the use of coconut oil particularly. Nearly 90 per cent of the fat in coconut oil is saturated fat. Many food products are made with coconut oil, including artificial milks, cream substitutes, and the fats used in bakery goods, cookies, plus innumerable prepared foods. Often on the label, coconut oil travels under the disguise "vegetable oil," a term that covers a multitude of sins. Don't accept this term as an indication of the nature of the fat ingredient in a prepared food.

There are a number of problems people have in following a healthy diet because of various health situations. Many of these can be circumvented with a little planning. High on the list are the large number of adults who have very low tolerance for the milk sugar lactose. This limits how effectively they can use dairy products. Since the intolerance is usually not 100 per cent, many of these people can tolerate small amounts of dairy products, but probably not enough to meet their daily calcium needs. These individuals can use a substitute for milk products. Perhaps some of the best ones are those milk substitutes prepared for babies who have an allergy or lactose intolerance problems. These can usually be found in the baby-food section of most supermarkets.

There are also some adult milk substitutes. Be sure, however, to use those made of soybean products or some products other than coconut oil. If you are using a milk substitute made with coconut oil, you may be significantly increasing the amount of saturated fat in your diet. This can increase the likelihood of developing atherosclerosis. Some of the health food stores also have cans of powdered soybean milk preparations which can be used as substitutes for milk. Both the baby-food milk substitutes and the soybean powdered milk substitutes have been designed to replace milk. If you look at the list of ingredients, most will show amounts of calcium and protein similar to ordinary milk. There is some variation in the calcium content in some of these different products, so it pays to check the label.

Still another approach to the milk-intolerance problem is to include in the diet other foods rich in calcium. These are listed in the discussion on calcium. Also, don't forget hard water may be an important additional source of calcium.

Some individuals do not tolerate gluten. Specifically, it causes them to have severe bouts of diarrhea with problems of absorbing anything from the small intestine. This can lead to multiple vitamin deficiencies and even destruction of the normal enzyme systems that enable absorption of ordinary sugar as well as the milk sugar lactose. This is a very serious problem because it strikes at a basic source of the vitamin B group. The gluten protein is found in all cereals, other than corn and rice, and all foods that contain cereal products. Individuals with this problem will have trouble consuming cold cuts because many contain cereal. Even commercial ice cream may be made with flour. Innumerable prepared foods must be excluded from the diet.

These rare individuals are a good example of those who can profit from the use of vitamin pills. These people have a medical problem that makes it impossible for them to have a normal diet. They can use enriched rice and corn products, which are commonly enriched with the vitamin-B-complex group, as their bread substitute. Cornmeal is also useful, but many cornbread mixes contain wheat flour and hence gluten. By using enriched rice and corn products, and obtaining vitamins in vegetables and fruits, it's possible to meet the vitamin-B-complex requirements. This requires a great deal of juggling, so it might be wise to take vitamin B complex regularly.

Very few people cannot tolerate fruits and vegetables. There may be selective problems for one or more fruits or vegetables that an individual can't tolerate, but almost always other items in this group can be used. For this reason, no recommended substitutions for this group are needed. Don't forget that fruits are an important source of potassium.

Some individuals need to restrict their salt. The restriction usually won't need to be any more severe than simply not including salt in cooking or adding salt at the table. If it's necessary to limit salt even more strictly than this, the milk and meat group, particularly, may have to be limited. This requires extra attention to obtain adequate amounts of good protein and calcium on such a diet. Rice, of course, is a low-salt food, and enriched rice helps to provide vitamins, but it's low in protein. High on the list of foods which can be included for individuals with these problems are the mature bean seeds, particularly soybeans. Unsalted, dry-roasted soybeans would provide a valuable protein source in the diet without significantly increasing the sodium intake. Such individuals may also profit from the use of protein powders.

Whenever sodium restriction needs to be this severe, the person will have to be under a doctor's constant supervision, and through the advice of the doctor and employing the general principles mentioned here, it should be possible to provide the kind of diet that would meet the daily needs. And, of course, when a medical condition warrants it, there's no reason vitamin supplements or the protein powders shouldn't be used.

Finally, some individuals will need to make extra efforts to provide sufficient iron in the diet, despite iron-enriched bread and other enriched products. Those who have this problem can increase the amount of those food items listed as rich sources of iron (see the chapter on iron). If the iron requirement still cannot be met, an iron supplement might need to be utilized, as recommended by the patient's doctor. This is particularly true of women during their menstruating years, especially if they tend to have heavy menstrual flow.

The listing of foods within the basic four food groups only tells you what you need to do to meet your protein, vitamin, and mineral requirements. It does not tell you how much food you need to satisfy your calorie requirements. Having sufficient calories in the diet is just as important to a well-balanced diet as having sufficient protein, vitamins, and minerals. Remember that calories, not vitamins, are the source of energy. The calorie needs will depend on each individual's living habits, including levels of physical activity and age. An infinite variety of food can be added to the diet to meet calorie needs. That is not the usual problem. The person who uses a lot of calories every day can get by with using empty-calorie foods, such as lard and sugar. If you need to restrict calories, you should meet the basic essentials listed above and then, if there's still any room left to use additional calories in the diet, you can add concentrated fats (oils and the like) and carbohydrates (sugars, syrups, and the like).

The additional calories can come from any of the items on the basic-four food lists, including vegetables, meat, milk, cereals, breads, or fruits. Remember, if you don't have enough calories in your diet, the important protein sources in your diet will be used for calories rather than being available for the building process for body regeneration and the formation of vital body substances, including those important hormones. Sufficient calories are protein spares making it possible to use the proteins for building substances instead of energy.

A number of rules have been formulated as to how many calories a person needs. They can only be a general guide, since the only important figure is how many calories you or members of your family need. You can tell whether you're getting enough calories or not by your energy level and by the presence of body fat. If you're restricting your calorie intake and you feel tired, it's likely you need more calories. Increased amounts of fat deposits you can feel or see underneath the skin indicate you're getting more calories than you need. Once you've eliminated excess fat stores, your best rule of thumb is your energy level.

38

UNDERNUTRITION ROBS YOUR ENERGY

When there's not enough food for the body, there's not enough energy. Not only will a person feel tired, but many of the body's vital functions are decreased or shut down because of an energy crisis. If you are tempted to go on a diet to lose weight, keep in mind that you may have an energy crisis.

A starting place to understand what really happens in the course of diets is to understand what happens to the human body during starvation. One of the earlier studies of the effects of complete starvation on man was carried out by F. G. Benedict in 1915. A thirty-one-day fast caused a loss of 29 pounds (13.2 kilograms). Keep this figure in mind because it means the fasting subject lost an average of a pound a day. Fasting episodes are not innocuous. A case in point is Terrance MacSwiney, the Mayor of Cork. In 1920 he fasted for seventy-four days, in the aftermath of the Irish troubles, until his death. In 1963 a pilot and his passenger survived a crash in the Canadian wilderness. They were lost for seven weeks. They had meager food supplies for one week and were without food for the ensuing six weeks. There are numerous examples of death from fasting for a period of four to five weeks. Many individuals, however, survive fasts for longer periods of time while under careful medical supervision. Some people have fasted over two hundred days, losing a third to a half pound a day.

In case you're tempted to try it, let me say unequivocally that I do not recommend fasting and consider it life-threatening. No one should be on a fasting diet program or a significantly reduced calorie intake unless under careful medical supervision. Even some of these circumstances are none too safe in the current day of diet fads and reducing gimmicks.

Even when the body receives no food, there is an expenditure of around 1500 to 2000 calories a day. The number of calories used depends on whether a person is totally or moderately inactive. Obviously, the less activity there is the fewer calories are used. This means that even on a zero calorie intake you can't expect to lose more than one-half to two-thirds pound of fat a day. There are 3500 calories in a pound of body fat. Obviously, a half pound of fat then contains 1750 calories, about enough to supply energy for a person who remains relatively inactive. The principle source of calories during fasting is the fat depots. If for any reason a person starts using muscle tissue as well, large weight losses can be achieved because there are only 600 calories in a pound of lean muscle. No health-minded individual, however, advocates losing large amounts of body protein, either from muscles or vital organs.

At the beginning of the fast, there is an initial loss of protein. This is apparently the fluid protein that's not already locked into a structured system or a part of a hormone or enzyme. After the first few days of the fast, less protein is used for body energy. In the Benedict studies, 7 to 8 grams of nitrogen continued to be lost throughout the thirty-one-day period. Now, if you'll recall, a gram of nitrogen is equated to 6.25 grams of protein in food. You can apply this same principle to body proteins since they're not really any different. Meat is meat, whether it's ours or some other mammal's. Seven to 8 grams of nitrogen lost from the body a day, then, is equivalent to about 45 to 50 grams of body protein. Other studies have provided slightly different figures, but the range is from 35 to 70 grams of protein a day.

If you want to translate this into muscle tissue, there are about 6 grams of protein in an ounce of muscle tissue, or 20 grams of protein for 100 grams of muscle tissue. (I use 6 grams here rather than 5, basing the weight on separable lean of muscle tissue. For food, the flesh usually contains more fat and, hence, less protein. Even lean fish often contain less protein in an ounce. For the entire meat-poultry-fish food group, I use 5 grams as an average value.) Forty-five grams of protein, then, is what you might expect in 225 grams or 7½ ounces of muscle tissue. Using weight-loss figures from the Benedict studies, during a thirty-one-day fast an individual would be losing on the average of a half pound of fat and a half pound of muscle each day. This would be a one pound weight loss daily for the thirty-one-day period, representing about 2000 calories a day. This is in keeping with the amount of muscle-mass loss individuals have after prolonged periods of starvation. The marked wasting of the body is not simply because fat depots are eliminated, but also because protein stores are lost.

Some investigators have suggested that the loss of protein during starvation might not be so great based on the observation of a loss of only 4 to 5 grams of nitrogen a day. Whether or not these figures include sources of nitrogen loss other than that included in measurements of urine samples is not so clear. But even with these small losses, you are still talking about a loss of 25 to 30 grams of protein or approximately 5 ounces (150 grams) of muscle tissue daily. So we're still in the neighborhood of losing a third of a pound of muscle mass daily on a starvation diet, even using the most optimistic measurements.

As soon as the starvation process begins, the energy system starts shutting down. You can measure this by seeing the decrease in oxygen consumption by the body. In the laboratory this translates into a decreased basal metabolic rate. It's really fairly simple. If you are not going to be processing as much food and extracting the energy from it, you won't need the oxygen for the processing system. The body temperature falls along with this because a part of processing food to energy is associated with generating heat.

Even at the onset of starvation, significant medical problems can occur. When there's not enough carbohydrate in the diet, the body initially loses salt, and with it goes water. The salt and water loss at the onset of starvation can cause a dramatic weight loss in some individuals. This is not necessarily good. It means there'll be less than an optimal amount of water in the tissues, and there won't be enough water in the blood. In short, such individuals become like a wilted plant that hasn't been watered adequately for several days. The loss of salt and water increases the sense of fatigue. It causes still another problem, a tendency to faint. There's less blood, and as soon as the individual stands up it will pool in the legs and lower part of the body.

Faintness, dizziness, and related symptoms are a characteristic of the initial salt and water loss that occurs at the onset of starvation. These symptoms are closely akin to those I observed in healthy young men at bed rest. We used bed rest to find out what weightlessness would do to our first astronauts. Bed rest, even if a person is eating a normal diet, results in loss of salt and water and a tendency to fainting. This has indeed been a complication of prolonged space flight. How severe it is varies a great deal. This is one explanation why people who are lying in bed for a day or two feel faint when they first get up. So whether it's bed rest or lack of carbohydrate in the diet, salt and water loss will occur, and with it circulation problems and a tendency to faint. In addition, the starvation diet can cause headaches and even mild nausea.

Certain cells in the body, including the brain cells and parts of the bone marrow, require glucose. Some investigators state that eventually some of the brain cells can adapt to using some fatty acids for energy, but others still require some glucose for their activity. The body is highly successful in maintaining the critical level of blood-glucose concentration for days of prolonged fasting. There are several ways this is done, even though there is no food, and hence no carbohydrates. The first two days the liver glycogen stores will be converted and used as blood glucose. Thereafter, other mechanisms may be employed. One of the principal ones is gluconeogenesis. You'll recall this means new formation of glucose from certain amino acids. This process tends to accelerate the depletion of the body proteins. Even the most optimistic studies show a consistent use of at least small amounts of body protein (perhaps as much as a third of a pound of body tissues or 30 grams of protein) to help provide the vital amount of glucose for those cells in the body that require it. The glucose for your brain literally comes from your muscles. This is one good biological example where muscle power means brain power. Remember that 100 grams of protein produce about 58 grams of blood glucose. A third of a pound of muscle tissue provides a minimum of 30 grams of protein, to be converted into 18 grams of blood glucose.

The reports to the public about fats being converted to glucose are confusing. In fact, fatty acids cannot be converted to blood glucose, but the glycerol part of fat (triglyceride) stored in the fat cells can. As a guide to this, the glycerol in 100 grams of fat can be converted into 12 grams of blood glucose. It doesn't take a mathematical genius to realize that a little less than a half pound of body fat (about 200 grams) will yield 24 grams of blood glucose. Add this to the 18 grams of blood glucose obtained from the breakdown of body protein, and you see where the body still gets more than 40 grams of glucose a day. This is probably sufficient to meet the needs of those vital cells which must use glucose in their metabolic functions.

There are still other ways to conserve glucose when you need to which are more complicated and probably not as important as the use of glycerol and conversion of amino acids to glucose.

While fasting, it is still necessary to provide a minimal amount of energy for the body, or those nearly 2000 calories the body still needs. The vast majority of these come from the mobilized fat depots. The liver doesn't have time to completely metabolize fatty acids while it's busily converting amino acids to glucose and juggling all the other stresses imposed on it during starvation. As a result, it forms a lot of acetoacetic acid or ketone bodies. You remember, the liver can't process ketone bodies to release energy. These must leave the liver and are circulated to the muscles and other organs of the body for use. They are run through the energy circle to release energy for the body's function.

During starvation a person shifts over to depending primarily on fat as a source of energy. This is a thought to keep in mind. Whenever you cut your calories appreciably, you're increasing the percentage of fat to provide calories for your body. Mobilizing the fat and using it in this way is not greatly different from eating a high-fat diet.

During starvation there are commonly more ketone bodies formed than are completely utilized. But, at the most, only about 20 grams of ketones are lost in the body in this way. This includes those lost in urine, which is often much less than 20 grams, and the insignificant amount lost in the breath as acetone. The 20 grams of ketone bodies can account for only about 100 calories. It follows, then, on a relatively solid chemical basis, that the loss of ketones during starvation is not an important mechanism for the weight loss that occurs.

The ketosis in starvation is not as bad as that in uncontrolled severe diabetics. Because diabetics are not getting or using insulin properly, even the glucose manufactured from glycerol and amino acids may not be used properly. Also, look again at your metabolic map. Note that the processing of active acetate around the energy circle requires OAA from glucose. If the cells can't use glucose and can't provide enough OAA, there will be trouble in processing acetic acid to energy. It is not surprising, then, that the acetic acid units are converted to ketone bodies. These and other problems cause an enormous buildup in ketone bodies which leads to chemical imbalances, coma, and even death, if not corrected.

The problems associated with starvation don't end with the simple ones I've mentioned. Actually, there is a tendency for more fat to be mobilized in the fatty tissues than the liver is able to process. Under normal circumstances, the liver is designed to process carbohydrates as well as fats. When it must process fats alone and is overloaded, fat globules begin to accumulate in the liver, producing fatty liver. This can lead to scarring and serious damage to the liver itself.

Prolonged fasting tends to mobilize bone calcium. More calcium is lost in the urine because of the acid ketone bodies generated during starvation. Over long periods of time this can lead to significant softening of the bones and other medical disorders.

The problems of the skeleton are not usually considered a major problem in starvation because death develops before changes have advanced to the state to cause significant difficulties with the skeleton. It is, however, important in young growing people because the first stage in bone formation and skeletal development is the laying down of important proteins. These later become calcified. If starvation occurs during the growth period, there will be a decreased rate of growth. If this is not corrected before the growth phase has completed its cycle, stunted growth can result.

Although starvation is a serious problem, it's not one that most of us are likely to experience, but a large portion of our population is constantly exposed to serious undernutrition. This is particularly true with diet fads advertised to induce weight loss. High on the list of these are the low-carbohydrate diets and *Dr. Atkins' Diet Revolution.* Considering these diets, it's well to recall the experiments that have already been done on undernutrition. In one study of twelve healthy subjects accustomed to having 3100 calories a day, their diet intake was reduced to 1600 to 1800 calories for a period of five weeks. During this period these subjects lost 10 per cent of their body weight.

Later these subjects were allowed to increase their intake to almost 2000 calories a day, still well below their customary calorie intake. They were maintained on this diet for a period of months. Although their body weight stabilized, they continued to experience considerable deterioration in body function. In plain language, they were weak and tired all the time. That's not surprising. The amount of energy available from the diet simply wasn't adequate for the young subjects.

In addition, they lost their sex drive. Incidentally, undernourished women tend to stop having menstrual periods and have sexual difficulties as well. The subjects had serious mental changes, including depression and withdrawal from any forms of activity. These changes accompanied the general shutdown in the energy system, a mechanism designed by nature to protect the body during periods of nutritional deprivation.

In a similar study, Ancel Keys of the University of Minnesota studied the effects of a 1570-calorie diet in thirty-two healthy young adults who ordinarily ate approximately 3500 calories a day. These individuals were kept on their diet for twenty-four weeks. They weren't bad diets, either, since they contained 50 to 55 grams of protein, 30 to 45 grams of fat, and 300 grams of carbohydrate. The diets weren't low in carbohydrates as occurs with some popular fad diets, and even the protein intake exceeded current RDA values. These healthy young people on this degree of calorie restriction lost 25 per cent of their original body weight. Incidentally, they were supplied with ample vitamins and minerals to be sure they didn't develop any vitamin or mineral deficiencies.

The young subjects experienced the kind of physical changes you would expect to see with severe weight loss. The face appeared wasted and emaciated. The skin was usually cold and even slightly bluish, which we call cyanosis. The hair tended to grow slowly and even fall out in large amounts. The fingernails also grew slowly. These things all depend on the formation of new protein. Cuts and wounds tended to heal more slowly. These individuals were cold all the time, even when the temperature was warm. Associated with the total decrease in the metabolic function as the energy system was shut down, there was less need for transporting oxygen. It's not surprising then that the heart rate slowed to levels as low as thirty-five beats a minute. There were, of course, the symptoms of faintness and giddiness associated with the loss of water, salts, and minerals from the body. This in turn led to muscle cramps.

There were marked changes in psychological behavior with a sharp decrease in spontaneous activities and a general tendency to withdraw. There were decreased functions of the endocrine glands and generalized symptoms of indigestion causing feelings of gassiness, colic, and diarrhea. About the only good thing that could be said to have occurred during the study was that the sensation of hunger disappeared after the first few days of the study. This is common in the presence of semistarvation, and since these individuals were taking carbohydrates, these classic studies demonstrate that you do not have to eliminate carbohydrates entirely to have a loss of appetite in the presence of undernutrition.

The problems that occurred during the twenty-four weeks of undernutrition didn't stop after returning to a normal diet. Another thought to keep in mind if you want to go on a severe calorie-restricted diet is that these previously healthy young subjects continued to feel tired and had a loss of sex drive with other manifestations of low energy level for some time after the diet. A six-month period of normal living with a superhigh calorie intake and rehabilitation was necessary to return these individuals to the level of energy and physical capacity they enjoyed prior to the undernutrition period.

These studies demonstrate conclusively that our metabolic processing system requires a certain amount of energy to function properly. This energy must be provided by food. While energy stores are present in fat, it's not always easy to get it all mobilized. It's wise to be careful about calorie restriction if you want to avoid the adverse effects documented in the presence of starvation and undernutrition. These thirty-two healthy young adults were on a diet of approximately 1600 calories a day. You can appreciate then why a 1000- or 1200-calorie diet is sheer folly for most normal active adults.

39

THOSE FAD WEIGHT-REDUCING
METHODS CAN BE A DRAG

Nothing demonstrates the public's preoccupation with being overweight so much as the recurrent enthusiasm for reducing diets and other weight-reducing fads. A high proportion of the population in industrialized nations have good reason to be preoccupied with obesity, since it is often a major health hazard. The reasons for being concerned about obesity are more often related to physical appearance than health considerations. The association of slimness with youthfulness is a major factor.

The public gullibility for weight-loss gimmicks is indicative of the recurrent desire to get something for nothing. This is the basic reason for the astonishing popularity of diet programs, such as *Dr. Atkins' Diet Revolution*, which promises to give you the capacity to "stay thin forever" while eating as much as you want, or its remarkably similar predecessor, *Calories Don't Count*. The latter led its author, Dr. Herman Taller, into legal difficulties.

It's true you can lose weight on many of these diet fads, but weight loss alone is not necessarily desirable, as you have seen from the results of starvation and undernutrition. If weight loss alone were the only goal, you could solve that problem with an advanced case of tuberculosis, disseminated cancer, or uncontrolled diabetes. Your doctor understands very well how to induce weight loss. The problem is to induce weight loss while preserving the health of the individual.

Not all of the popularized concepts are bad in all instances. Under careful medical supervision, individuals who are grossly obese can gain certain advantages by using some of these principles. They become dangerous, however, when carried out as a do-it-yourself project without adequate or competent medical supervision.

The low-carbohydrate, high-protein diets are nothing new. They have been recycled with various modifications for years. Perhaps the first of these was the Banting diet used by William Banting in 1863. The diet was prescribed for him by Dr. William Harvey, and it had a startling effect in reducing his corpulent frame. The diet was really a low-calorie diet, not just a low-carbohydrate diet. Although it restricted sweets and starches, it did include vegetables, which are carbohydrates.

Many of the advocates of the low-carbohydrate diet begin with the idea that early man did not consume carbohydrates; hence, man was genetically not geared to processing carbohydrates. As I mentioned earlier, this theme was echoed in both *Calories Don't Count* and *Dr. Atkins' Diet Revolution* and is equally wrong in both instances. The facts are that early man depended heavily on carbohydrates and large portions of the world today still obtain over 80 per cent of their calories from carbohydrates. In certain parts of Asia as much as 95 per cent of the calories in the diet are from carbohydrate sources. In these parts of the world such things as "low blood sugar," obesity, and heart and vascular disease are of little or no significance.

Most of the earlier low-carbohydrate diets recommended included a small amount of carbohydrates in the diet, usually 40 to 60 grams. This was included in order to prevent ketosis, the problem of producing ketone bodies as a result of processing body fat and protein without carbohydrates. This small amount may be useful, and some authorities claim that it's sufficient to avoid protein loss seen in starvation or no-carbohydrate situations. The Atkins' diet went one step further. Atkins recommended starting the diet "with a daily intake of zero grams of carbohydrates," and maintaining the diet thereafter below 40 grams of carbohydrate a day. He wanted the diet to cause ketosis.

Although even reducing carbohydrate intake significantly can contribute to loss of salt and water, a total interdiction of carbohydrate is almost certain to induce this effect. This indeed will cause a dramatic initial decrease in pounds from dehydration, but not from loss of body fat deposits. It is the gimmick of sudden water loss with low-carbohydrate, high-protein diets which causes many dieters to think they're having a striking success. This initial water loss will last just as long as the person stays on the diet. As soon as a properly nutritious diet is resumed, including carbohydrates, salt and water will be retained to the levels necessary for optimal health. Those dramatic 5- and 10-pound losses the first week are mostly fluid, not fat. No wonder a number of people who try these diets experience faintness, weakness, dizziness, and fatigue, often accompanied by nausea. These are the symptoms you see at the onset of starvation.

Almost all of these diets work because they really decrease the calorie intake. It may be true, as Dr. Atkins claims, that you can eat all you want and stay slim forever, but the gimmick is you won't want to eat very much. Ketosis and associated chemical changes result in loss of appetite. The usual hunger-type response you're prone to experience if you're not eating enough isn't there. The nausea and accompanying complaints that some have may well be related to liver dysfunction. After all, high-fat diets, and that's what you're on if you're depending on a lot of the fat stores from the body to provide calories, lead to fatty deposits in the liver. This has a lot to do with how the alcoholic develops liver disease.

Many of the foods on such diets classified as high-protein foods are really low-calorie foods. A good example is lean round steak. It takes a full pound of the separable lean of raw round steak to provide 600 calories. That means you could eat 32 ounces a day and still get only 1200 calories. This is because the meats are about 70 per cent water. The same concept applies to fish and chicken. Thus, lean meats, fish, and chicken are all relatively low-calorie items and serve to fill you up without adding a lot of calories to your diet. There is nothing wrong with using these items on a weight-control program, but these normally good foods should not be used to exclusion of other needed nutrients in the diet.

Even Atkins acknowledges that most people on his diet get fewer calories and, as he states, "Most people eat less, but it's only because what they get on this diet so completely satisfies their hunger. They find they just can't eat as much as they used to." And Atkins goes on to say, "I don't expect that most of you will feel like making this much of a production of meal preparation every day. You may well be quite contented most of the time with meat, chicken, or fish with a salad for lunch and dinner." All of which means these individuals are on a low-calorie diet. What's worse, if you don't stay on these diets you usually tend to gain the weight right back. Particularly during the weight gain, there may be an increase in fatty particles and cholesterol in the bloodstream. This contributes, especially in susceptible individuals, to the risk of atherosclerosis and heart disease. Even Atkins admits, in reference to his own diet, "I concede that the worst feature about this diet is the rapidity with which you gain if you abandon it."

There will not be any miraculous weight loss because calories are washed out in the form of ketone bodies. As I mentioned in the discussion on the formation of ketone bodies, during absolute starvation you can't count on losing more than 100 calories a day as ketones. This includes the ketone bodies washed out by the kidneys and the bad breath from acetone. Since there are 3500 calories in a pound of fat, it's not likely that a great number of pounds of fat are going to be lost quickly at this rate.

The weight of evidence seems to be that in most instances what success does occur from the low-carbohydrate diets, including Doctor Atkins' program, is a direct result of a reduction in calorie intake. Contrary to public claims that you don't need to consider calories, the truth is this is the basis for any success achieved by these diets. The idea that "the old calorie counting system doesn't work" is completely without scientific basis and borders on fraud.

In addition to the problems related to undernutrition, some other hazards can be incurred by the low-carbohydrate diets. Many of these so-called low-carbohydrate, high-protein diets are really high-fat diets. Dr. Atkins compounds this problem by advocating the use of large amounts of eggs and high-cholesterol foods. Such a diet is thought by many serious scientists to be a significant factor in increasing the likelihood of atherosclerosis. In one experiment subjects on an all-meat diet developed visible fat within the blood itself, and their cholesterol rose to levels as high as 800. The metabolic machinery must process the fat in your food plus the fat from your body stores. The combined results mean an enormous portion of your calories comes from fat.

It may be true that during the period of weight loss a number of subjects do have a temporary decrease in their cholesterol level. Just decreasing the calories enough to induce weight loss means that a greater portion of the active acetate on your metabolic map will be processed by the energy circle and used for energy. This means there will be less available along the line to be processed to form cholesterol. But once the weight has stabilized and a person has adjusted to a new lower calorie intake and a major portion of that calorie intake is fat, there's likely to be a significant increase in blood fat and cholesterol levels.

One of the more popular diet fads is the "Stillman diet," sometimes called the "water diet." It is reported that over five million of these diet books have been snapped up by weight-conscious Americans. It too is a low-carbohydrate diet. How dangerous this diet can be is underscored by a recent study by scientists at Peter Bent Brigham hospital and Harvard Medical School in Boston, reported in the April 1, 1974, issue of the *Journal of the AMA*. Dr. Frank Rickman and others who conducted the study of the Stillman diet reported that the diet caused an average increase of 16 per cent in the blood cholesterol level in the dieting subjects. The study was continued only a short time but illustrates the effect these so-called low-carbohydrate diets can have on blood cholesterol levels. This is particularly dangerous if continued any length of time in middle-aged men who are already prone to heart and vascular disease. Incidentally, the subjects had the weakness, fatigue, and other problems of diets that overly restrict carbohydrates. The real hazards imposed by these dietary methods have been rather well documented.

Once the enthusiasm for a fad diet wears off and an individual returns to his previous eating habits, during the period of weight gain there's apt to be a significant and dangerous rise in the blood fat and cholesterol levels. No one should be on a low-carbohydrate program without being monitored by a competent physician and laboratory at frequent intervals, in terms of the blood cholesterol.

The high-fat diet associated with a number of these programs, and the utilization of body fat in addition, may overload the liver with fat particles and lead to fatty liver and liver damage. This is particularly bad in starvation because of the absence of some of the protective lipotropic factors I discussed. It's probably true, then, that the person who is on a low-carbohydrate diet, which includes considerable meat, may be better protected than the individual undergoing starvation. But remember, an excessively high-fat diet alone may contribute to a fatty liver.

If one is to achieve success and "stay thin forever," it will be necessary to stay on these particular diets forever, unless you want to learn something about nutrition and do it the sensible way. Then there is the long-term, adverse effect of loss of calcium. The formation of ketone bodies and the disturbed chemistry contributes to this problem. The loss of calcium on a long-term basis can lead to softening of the bones. A high percentage of women have a buffalo hump or dowager's hump and increased susceptibility to fractures after the menopause. This is worse on a calcium-deficient diet. Many authorities feel you can significantly decrease the likelihood of middle age softening of the bone by increasing the amount of calcium in the diet. In any case, the Atkins diet and many other low-carbohydrate diets are deficient in calcium, since milk is reasonably rich in carbohydrates and cannot be used in the amounts needed to meet the calcium demands.

Of course, many of these diets, specifically including the Atkins diet, are grossly deficient in vitamins. The elimination of vegetables and cereals, which are important carbohydrate sources as well as vitamin and mineral sources, makes this inevitable. In fact, Dr. Atkins belongs to the supervitamin group and has advocated large doses of vitamins along with his vitamin-deficient ketone-body-forming diet. It would seem wiser to eat a diet that provides all of nature's vitamins in the food. You may solve the problem of the known deficiencies by pills, but one can't help but wonder about the unknown deficiencies that aren't defined. Surely we don't know everything yet.

It should be mentioned that along with *Calories Don't Count, Dr. Atkins' Diet Revolution, The Drinking Man's Diet,* and other versions of low-carbohydrate high-protein diets, that the addition of drinking large amounts of water doesn't alter the basic chemical facts. The addition of this ingredient just increases the necessity to stay close to the bathroom.

The low-carbohydrate diets and any of the crash diet programs, including fasting, have in common the danger of precipitating an acute attack of gout. This can occur even in a person who is not ordinarily susceptible to gout. The destruction of body tissues releases nucleic acids. These can be metabolized to uric acids and cause a sharp rise of the uric-acid concentration in the body. This can cause uric-acid crystals to form in the joints. The next thing you know the individual who started out on a diet to lose weight ends up with a red, hot, swollen toe with a typical case of the gout.

Weight reduction is desirable in people who have gout or for anyone who is significantly overweight. An acute attack of gout is an example of too much too soon, or the crash weight-loss approach. It's just another reason why programs have to be sensible and carried out on a gradual basis.

Closely related to some of the diet fads is the concept of administering small amounts of thyroid to individuals who are overweight. It's correct to give thyroid to stimulate the metabolic process in individuals who truly have a low thyroid function. More often than not, individuals who are significantly overweight do not have abnormally low thyroid function. The net result of giving these individuals thyroid is that their normal thyroid function is depressed. As I have mentioned, the total amount of the thyroid from the pill and that formed by the depressed thyroid gland just about equals the amount of thyroid hormone before anyone interfered with the process.

There may be a need for thyroid replacement in middle and later years. Studies show that a number of individuals do have a slowdown in thyroid function in later years. The mechanisms are not entirely clear, but it is part of the aging process. Before giving thyroid, though, the doctor will usually want to know what the actual status of thyroid function is. As I mentioned earlier, if a person is taking thyroid needlessly, when it is stopped there will be a period of fatigue. This is the time lag required for the thyroid to resume normal function. It does not mean that there was low thyroid function to begin with.

In the past, there has been an unscrupulous practice of giving magic pills which contain small amounts of thyroid, medicines of the speed group such as dexedrine or amphetamine, used to suppress the appetite, and a diuretic to wash out salt and water. Sometimes these even contained digitalis, a powerful heart stimulant. Washing out water and salt, whether by a starvation diet, a low-carbohydrate diet, or a pill, is not a means of eliminating body fat unless the individual becomes so ill from such unethical treatments that weight loss results from illness. Moreover, some of these potent combinations of pills have caused death. This kind of pill has no place in weight reduction.

Appetite-suppressing pills perhaps have some use under controlled circumstances, at least to motivate the person to start on a diet. Many of them, though, are dangerous and in general shouldn't be recommended. They often cause nervousness and other problems which are worse than obesity. Some of the more dangerous ones have already been removed from the market.

Included in the pill group are laxatives. Some of the readers of my syndicated column have sent me advertisements from popular newspapers which I consider unethical. They promise enormous weight loss within a few days after taking pills. Some of the individuals who have taken these preparations have reported marked diarrhea with severe illness. You should avoid all the advertised weight-reducing regimes. Almost without exception, these are methods which would be considered unethical by knowledgeable scientists and reputable physicians.

Beyond the tablets and diets are other gimmicks for weight loss, including sweat belts, sweat pants, and numerous devices designed to cause the body to lose water. You can do the same thing with a heat cabinet, and the body weight loss is water and salt. A lot of the weight a football player loses on a hot Saturday afternoon is water and salt. Coaches know this and try to replace this during the game because they recognize that this loss can be damaging to the athlete's topnotch performance. This is no less true of the rest of us. Any of the devices which cause excessive loss of salt and water is apt to disturb our chemistry in such a way as to produce significant problems. Heat treatments, belts, and the like, then, as far as loss of actual pounds of fat are concerned, are all gimmicks.

Most individuals who feel an urge to lose a few pounds, or even a lot of pounds, are ready victims for the exaggerated claims that are ever-present in our news media. With the age- and weight-conscious nature of our society, the overweight person is a ready target for these devices. Having repeatedly seen the effects and failures of most of these programs on a do-it-yourself basis, the best recommendation I can give is not to begin any significant weight-reduction program that does not have the approval of your physician. Avoid at all costs a crash program. Most individuals do not become obese overnight, and they cannot safely reduce their excess body weight in an overnight effort. In a sensible weight-control program there is no place for crash diets, fad diets, or crash exercise programs. What is needed is a sensible program of good nutrition and living habits to enable your metabolic system to provide optimal amounts of energy, proper cell-growth replacement, and the formation of normal hormones and enzymes. These are the things good health is made of.

40

SENSIBLE WEIGHT CONTROL TO PROTECT YOUR HEALTH AND ENERGY LEVEL

Is there a secret to preventing obesity? Yes, there is, and the facts have been around a long time. There is a lot more to preventing obesity than just "burning off calories" or starving yourself. If you understand this, you can eat a healthier diet that gives you more energy and still not get fat. For years people have been trying to lose weight by going on diets that are often not as good as the semistarvation diets that had such a bad effect on healthy subjects. No wonder these efforts have been such a big flop. The other approach has been to use the endurance exercises like running, jogging, or walking. These are all good, but you must do a lot of regular exercise to use many calories. I hope you won't misunderstand my point. I am all for good endurance exercises done properly, but they are not the sole key to preventing obesity.

The problem with most programs for the treatment of obesity is that they are not designed to treat the real cause. We have been engaged in "symptomatic treatment." If a person is too fat, the symptom is attacked by decreasing the amount he eats, rather than treating the underlying cause for the obesity. Obviously, once the symptomatic treatment is stopped the person gets fat again because the underlying problem has not been treated. This is the same thing that can happen if you give a person aspirin for a headache caused by a brain tumor. The aspirin can relieve the headache, but once its effects have worn off, the headache may return because the tumor is still there. Now, there has been remarkable success in treating some obesity problems. Those rare cases, and I do mean rare, of low thyroid function are helped with treatment and so are a few other rare cases, but the vast majority of people who have creeping obesity with increasing years get symptomatic treatment.

Some of the problems of obesity are indeed caused simply by overeating and eating the wrong things. These problems are greatly helped by a proper diet. In this case, the real cause is being treated. It may be necessary to look beyond overeating to find out why the person is overeating and what can be done about it. The fact remains that most people get fat while continuing to eat about the same things they ate in earlier years and while doing about the same amount of physical activity.

The real problem in most cases of obesity begins with how many calories you use while you are not doing anything, not while you are exercising. The calories you use at rest under standard conditions (the basal metabolism) decreases as you get older. This is a very important fact. It means simply that if you eat the same number of calories you ate when you were younger and do the same amount of physical activity, you will still get fat. Scientists have tended to ignore this obvious and important factor in the cause of obesity. The emphasis on calories eaten and the number used in physical activity has all but blinded us to the truth about most common problems of obesity, and particularly that middle-aged spread.

I've talked a lot about active cells as opposed to inactive cells in the body. The muscle cells are active cells. They are busy all the time, even when you are resting, and tend to process food around the energy circle to enable us to have more energy. The plain truth is that a heavy laborer or well-trained athlete does use more calories at rest than a sedentary individual at rest. The difference is important and significant in terms of obesity. Fat cells are fairly inactive. They don't have nearly as many blood vessels to them as do the active muscle cells. They are used mostly to store energy as fat and release it when we need it. Other than manipulating fat, they don't have a lot of metabolic activity and can get by on a lot less oxygen than our active muscle cells.

As we get older we tend to lose our muscle cells—we say our muscle mass decreases. There are many reasons for this, and certainly one of these is failure to maintain physical activity of the type that builds and strengthens muscles. Sex hormones are important. Male hormone tends to stimulate the formation of muscles, female hormones do not. I might add here that both sexes have some of both hormones. In the main, most exercise physiologists have tended to emphasize the calories used during physical activity while ignoring the decrease in calories used associated with decreased muscle mass.

Let's take a look at what really happens. A woman who is 65 inches tall and weighs 121 pounds can be used as an example. Under standard resting conditions for a period of twenty-four hours she will use the following number of calories at different age levels:

20 years	1382 calories
40	1363
45	1344
50	1325
55	1296
60	1267
65	1239
70	1229
75	1219

Women tend to plateau in their calorie needs at rest between the ages of twenty and forty years. It is after forty that the need for calories at rest begins to decrease sharply. This is the time the middle-aged spread is worst. At first glance you may not think that the decrease in calories used at rest between age twenty and fifty is that important, but remember this is day in and day out, 365 days a year. That decrease of 57 calories used a day represents the number of calories in 6 pounds of fat a year. Think what that means. If a woman at fifty continues the same patterns she had at twenty, she would be gaining 6 pounds of fat a year. To show you what happens in our standard woman, I have converted the decrease in her resting energy requirements into pounds of fat a year and it looks like this for each age group:

20 years	0.0 pounds of fat a year
40	2.0
45	4.0
50	6.0
55	9.0
60	12.0
65	15.0
70	16.0
75	17.0

The story is even worse for men. For a standard man, let's use a man 70 inches tall weighing 155 pounds. Common values for the calories used under standard resting conditions over twenty-four hours for such a healthy man at different age levels are:

20 years	1736 calories
25	1705
30	1661
35	1649
40	1649
45	1638
50	1627
55	1607
60	1593
65	1570
70	1537
75	1519

There is no twenty-year plateau in the use of calories in men as you see in women. There isn't a great change between thirty and forty years of age.

Men mature physically a bit slower than women, and for this reason we should use age twenty-five as representative of a physically mature person. By converting the changes in resting calorie requirements into pounds of fat a year, you get the following values for the different age groups:

25 years	0.0 pounds of fat a year
30	4.7
35	5.8
40	5.8
45	7.0
50	8.2
55	10.3
60	11.8
65	14.0
70	17.5
75	19.3

The only reason people don't become barely movable blimps of fat as they get older is that they don't continue to eat as much as they ate at younger ages. Then, too, they lose muscle mass. Often a man may weigh the same, but his measurements change. His waistline tends to get bigger than his chest measurement. Some have laughingly said to me that their chest had sunk. The loss of muscle and the gain of fat tends to balance out the effect. The result, of course, is that a much larger part of the body weight is fat, and that is not considered good for health. It certainly is not good for energy. Those active cells are the main source of producing the energy you need to keep you full of the zest for living. Forming fat doesn't provide you with any energy or zest. It doesn't generate any ATP.

You can look at this another way. A twenty-five-year-old standard man will use 186 more calories a day at rest than a seventy-five-year-old man of comparable height and weight. This means the seventy-five-year-old man will need to walk three miles a day just to use the same energy the young man uses resting. It's diabolical, but if you don't maintain enough active cells in the body, you will need to work harder and harder as you get older just to keep from getting fat.

These figures are also supported by studies done on Professor Magnus Levy, one of the pioneers in studying resting energy needs. He was studied by his methods in 1891 at the young age of twenty-six years, and again in 1941 at age seventy-six. As a young man, under standard resting conditions, he used 67 calories an hour. When he was seventy-six he only used 52 calories an hour. In other words, he used 360 calories a day more during standard resting conditions when he was young than he did fifty years later. Incidentally, he didn't get fat either, but he had to prevent this by not eating as much as he formerly did and by his living patterns. There is no other way. He had lost 16 pounds between ages twenty-six and seventy-six. No doubt this was part of the loss of his muscle mass.

Young children use even more calories at rest than young adults. During the growing phase they use a lot of calories in building new tissues. A ninety-year-old person uses less than two-thirds the calories a ten-year-old uses when you correct for the differences in body size.

The decrease in calorie need at rest with increasing age values I have listed are only a guide. Many people have even a greater decrease in resting calorie requirements. When this approaches a decrease of 500 calories a day, it is really a major factor. The failure to pay more attention to the changing resting calorie requirements has led to greater emphasis on calorie-expending exercises. You can think of the calorie balance problem as having three parts, not two. There is the point of how many calories you eat, calories in. Then, there are two ways calories are spent, calories out. One is by physical activity, and the other is the resting requirement. The resting requirement is literally the body's overhead. What is left is the profit and can be spent on activity. In many people, the overhead factor is the most important.

A man working in a sedentary office job may use 1500 calories a day as overhead or resting requirements and only 500 a day for physical activity. That's not much. While I agree it is important to improve the activity program and use more calories, the reason this man starts getting fat all at once is because his overhead requirements start going down, not because he has a further decrease in activity. Since the overhead of 1500 calories is the major way his body uses calories, we need to take a much better look at what we can do to maintain this level. In short, treat the real cause for this man's obesity. A proper treatment program should include measures to maintain the resting energy turnover by the body, an activity program to use excess calories, and a program to control the excess ingestion of calories.

There are probably a lot of factors related to how many active cells a person has other than just the muscle mass, but it is one of the most important factors. Even the amount of some of our important hormones are directly related to how much muscle mass the body has. I have emphasized this point because it has been too long neglected. Obviously, an important approach to the problem of obesity is to do what you can to maintain the use of calories at rest. This means trying to maintain our bodies so they are strong and have adequate muscles. It changes the emphasis from just hours of running to burn up calories to include those strength-type exercises that develop and maintain muscles.

It doesn't take very long to do strength-type exercises. You needn't become exhausted to build and maintain a suitable amount of muscle mass. In building and maintaining active cells, you may find you have a lot more energy and will feel more like doing your endurance exercises. Of course, running, jogging, and other endurance exercises also help to build muscle mass as well as use calories. They are very good, but you can also profit a great deal by the muscle-building programs to help keep you from getting fat. This is true for both men and women. If you avoid decreasing your resting energy needs, you will have taken an important step toward avoiding obesity. Exercises that help you build and maintain active cells, as well as use calories from the activity, can enable you to eat a more satisfying diet. You can also see from the above figures that the role of exercise in maintaining your health and in preventing obesity has really been short-changed. There is a lot more to exercise than just using calories during the physical activity. Good exercise programs build active cells and that will also make an important contribution to keeping you from falling into the fat and fatigued group.

One of the big problems with symptomatic treatment is that it can make matters worse. A major source of your energy is generated by those active cells. They are the ones that process foods around the energy circle. When they decrease in amount, your energy level falls. Those individuals with young vigorous bodies are not short on energy. This is not the time to cut back on your food to the point you decrease your available energy even more. You need to attack the cause and build up your body, not starve it. Severe diets often result in loss of active muscle cells. This is particularly true if the protein requirements are not met or the calorie intake is too low. Remember what happened to the young subjects in the Minnesota experiment on 1600 calories a day. Part of their loss of weight included loss of muscle mass. If you diet unwisely, you can decrease the number of active cells you have. That means your body is less capable of producing energy for you and your resting calorie requirement will go down. If that is already the underlying problem, you can see the treatment will actually make the problem worse.

Yes, you might lose weight while you are on the unsound diet, but afterward you will need to continue to cut back more on food if you have lost vital active cells and didn't replace them. Dieting isn't always the answer. You can see from this problem the importance of a combined exercise and diet program in combating or preventing obesity.

Of course, food intake is important in weight control. It remains true that the degree of obesity is directly related to the amount of food energy consumed and the amount of energy used. The only shift in emphasis I would like to make in this discussion is that the energy used isn't all just visible physical activity. A lot of the energy used depends on the fundamental life processes that are directly related to the amount of active cellular material in our bodies. One of the basic principles in preventing obesity should be directed toward maintaining a vigorous healthy body with an optimal amount of active cells.

The diet program used to prevent or correct obesity should be one that includes all the essential ingredients of a well-balanced diet. For this purpose you can consult the list of foods I have provided under the four basic food groups for a healthy diet. These should provide the skeleton for a weight-control diet. You can eat the proper amount of these and still only consume 1400 calories a day.

Using the basic food lists, you can construct your own diet. All you need to do is select the foods in each group that are lower in calories. Let's start with the milk group. You should choose four glasses of forti-fied skim milk a day (420 calories) or four glasses of buttermilk (360 calories). Of course, you could use some of each. This is a good start on your diet as you can meet your calcium requirements, get 0.4 milli-gram of your thiamine needs, and 1.0 milligram of riboflavin. Also, this will meet at least half of your protein requirements.

In the meat group choose the low-fat items. To help you in your choice and calorie calculation, use the separable lean of beef before preparing. On the average, 3½ ounces (100 grams) will provide 150 calories. Use fryer chicken and remove the skin before eating. A 5¼-ounce piece with bone will equal about 3½ ounces of flesh. The breast is the lowest-calorie piece. You can estimate that such a piece will yield 105 calories. To limit your fish serving use low-calorie fish or shellfish.

Low-Calorie Fish and Shellfish
75 to 125 Calories per 100 Grams (3½ Ounces)

Flounder	Pike
Catfish	Red Snapper
Cod	Tuna (fresh or water-pack)
Bass	Redfish
Haddock	Shrimp
Halibut	Drum
Clams	

Remember to rotate your meat dishes among these three groups—meat, fish, and poultry—and you will have an average of 240 calories for two such meat servings a day.

In the cereal group choose three (1 ounce, 28 grams) slices of bread (225 calories). You can splurge and include a cup of cooked oatmeal (130 calories).

Your choices from the fruit and vegetable group could be:

Calories in Some Fruits and Vegetables

Peas	58 calories per serving
Broccoli	27
Spinach	40
Green beans	30
Carrots	45
Grapefruit	44
Orange juice	36

Even if you use some sugar on your oatmeal and a dab of margarine on your bread, this plan would still be below 1400 calories. (The actual count is 1295 from the above figures). Of course, you don't have to stick to this exact plan. The beauty of the lists is that you can plan your own diet to suit your own taste. I don't advise trying to cut the calories down below the 1295 calories on this list. Remember that the starvation studies using 1600 calories a day caused a lot of problems. I would prefer that people used more calories and tried to lose weight very slowly. The foods you choose to add more calories to your diet are up to you. You would be wise, however, in choosing them to follow the recommendations of limiting your total fat, saturated-fat and cholesterol intake. Sweets do have some tendency to increase the formation of insulin. There may be some truth in the idea that this may contribute to using the fat path as opposed to the energy circle.

There are numerous ways individuals can plan the consumption of their calories for their diet program. One desirable system is to be on a relatively restricted intake one day and eat a normal, nutritious optimal diet on the second day. The second-day diet is equivalent to the diet one should stay on after the weight-loss program. This helps to establish dietary habits necessary to maintain optimal weight. Too often, after a specific dietary regime, people return to their old habits and regain the excess pounds.

Another approach is to make a limited reduction in the calories, not of sufficient degree to cause a major energy crisis, and stick to it longer while increasing your exercise level. The body will gradually eliminate excess fat deposits and achieve a new balance in line with your physical activity and dietary intake. If you do it properly and don't overdo the diet restriction, this will actually be a plus for your energy level.

Certain diet problems deserve special mention. Much of the problem of overeating is related to habits. At the beginning of your program, write down everything you eat every day, including each snack in the kitchen and every cocktail, as well as what you eat at the table. Look through the list and find out which ones aren't really necessary for your well-balanced diet, such as the sugar in the coffee, the spoonful of ice cream while you're dipping it out for the children, or that cocktail before dinner. Give some thought to why you eat, and identify the cues that cause you to reach for something. Often this is associated with social patterns. If you're eating because you're bored, try to do something about the boredom problem.

Many people eat because it's time to eat and behave like a Pavlovian dog when the bell rings. To solve this problem one needs to learn to eat because he is hungry and needs the food and not because of a time cue. If you're having trouble in adjusting your diet, it's sometimes not a bad idea to disrupt your usual mealtime sequence, if this is possible. Eat a half hour before your regular mealtime one day and a half hour later the next day. You can try eating earlier and decreasing the amount if you've been having an urge to eat far more than the calories you need on a well-balanced diet. Still another point is to try not to eat too fast. It takes about twenty minutes for the food you've eaten to start processes that signal the brain you've satisfied your hunger needs.

Once you've started on a diet, stick to it. Cheating on a diet is far more detrimental than most people realize. The stimulus that tells us we're hungry comes from a center in the brain. It's turned on to make us hungry when the blood glucose falls, then when enough glucose is present in the cells within the appetite center, it shuts off and our hunger stops. This center can be reset just as the thermostat in your house can be reset. To do this, though, requires a period of training it to a new level. Your appetite center is adjusted to being satisfied only when the blood-glucose level peaks. You'll have constant recurring hunger unless the blood-glucose level is constantly increased by eating. By eliminating sweets and concentrating on carbohydrates from cereal, vegetable, and fruit sources, these high peak levels of glucose can be eliminated and the appetite center will be reset at a lower level. This decreases the tendency to be hungry all the time.

The simple diet rules I have mentioned should be quite adequate for most people to prevent obesity. Remember, if you start showing any evidence of gaining weight, cut back on your calories a little, eliminating some of those items you don't need to provide the fundamental skeleton for the basic well-balanced diet. Then start increasing your level of physical activity. This includes attention to strength-type exercises to build up and maintain your muscle mass.

What about those unhappy people who want to gain weight? Can they do it by a special diet? It's not a very good idea. These people are geared to process more of their food around the energy circle. All that extra energy keeps them very active. After all, they are loaded with ATP. If they are successful in eating so many calories that they swamp their energy circle, the result is formation of fat via the fat path and cholesterol, not a good goal for health.

You can't increase the muscles and nonfat tissue by eating more protein, fat, or carbohydrate, or drinking alcohol. The only way you can have more muscles is to stimulate the body to alter its growth pattern. The simplest of these mechanisms is by the use of exercise. As the muscle is placed under load, as in weight lifting or by other means, it forms more creatine. This compound stimulates the growth of more muscle mass. Then you can lift more weight and form more creatine. Again, this stimulates the formation of more muscle mass and finally those muscles begin to bulge. These exercises are quite different from walking, jogging, running, and various endurance exercises. The endurance exercises do not progressively increase the tension load on a muscle. They are excellent for the heart and lungs, but to put meat on your bones there is no substitute for muscle-tensing and weight-lifting exercises. With the exercise to stimulate the growth of new muscles, you can then use part of those extra calories and protein in the building process. Otherwise the extra food is not going to do anything but generate fat.

The use of exercise in weight control has not received all the emphasis it deserves. Most of the emphasis has been on a calories-in, calories-out approach. This would suggest that it takes an awful lot of exercise to do anything about weight control. A 150-pound person walking one mile at a speed of three miles an hour will use only 60 calories more than he would while he was resting. Measurements of this sort have caused people to think that exercise has limited applications to weight control.

Walking is good exercise. It helps to maintain muscle mass, but it's not an ideal exercise for these purposes. You can use low-level endurance exercises, such as walking, to slowly burn off calories, but it's a painful and time-consuming procedure. You should think of exercise in two ways. One is the classic use to expend energy, and the other is exercise used to build up and maintain muscle mass, because this represents active cells. I am not suggesting it is necessary to build an enormous muscular development, but it is necessary to maintain a sufficient range of exercises to maintain the muscle mass as the years go by, pretty close to what it was during early adult physical maturity.

In the process of exercising a muscle, energy is used. At the same time the circulation is increased to deliver oxygen to the cells. All of this means that the metabolic processing unit primarily involves the use of the energy circle. If sufficient energy is used in this way, relatively little food energy will be left to take the fat path to energy storage. The increased circulation to the tissues may well enhance the continued use of the oxygen-dependent energy circle, releasing energy long after the initial exercise has stopped. Physiological studies have proved that increased oxygen consumption may continue for hours after increased physical activity has ceased.

The physical exercise may well act as a catalyst to the continued use of the energy path. If this is so, it means that more energy would be released to form ATP for bodily processes. This may be why the individual who engages in regular moderate amounts of physical activity always feels more energetic than the office worker who has been sitting quietly at a typewriter or involved in other sedentary activities all day. Exercise as a catalyst to the energy system may be far more important than the small number of calories used during physical activity.

Exercise cannot be used in weight control as a crash program any more than diets can be a crash program. It should be built into the daily life style of everyone. For best results, there should be frequent periods of physical activity throughout the day. This may be more important than distributing your food over several meals in a day, if you want to have a high energy level.

If you can do this comfortably without difficulty, you should gradually increase the walking period until you can comfortably walk three miles in one hour. Individuals who have not been moderately active physically shouldn't try to walk for a full hour or three miles initially. They should allow a period of several weeks to increase their exercise capacity to this level. Those who have been regularly physically active may not need to follow this precaution, but I consider it's better to do this if you are going to set up your own exercise program.

Once an individual has demonstrated that he can walk three miles in an hour without feeling tired, then he can consider more vigorous activity, whatever appeals to him—jogging, cycling, and other exercise activities. In general, I prefer for individuals who are going to increase their exercise level significantly above that involved in simple walking to have a medical evaluation and to discuss their exercise program with their doctor. Even so, if a 150-pound individual walks three miles a day regularly, in the course of a year he should use approximately the same amount of calories found in 18 pounds of fat. The key to a successful exercise program in the elimination and prevention of obesity is consistency.

From the facts about resting calorie needs and active cells, you can see that the most useful general calisthenic program is one that employs all the different muscles. It should include exercises that will use muscles through their full range of action. In addition, to maintain the muscle tone, most healthy individuals can profit from a sensible set of modified isometric exercises. These exercises should be done by beginning gradually from the toes to the head and contracting each set of muscles against each other. As an example, let's use the arm. If you contract the biceps and pull the fist up toward the shoulder and hold it steadily in this position, it will be an isometric contraction. Now, if you straighten the arm, moving the fist away from the shoulder, that would be an isotonic exercise. Keeping the arm muscles tense and moving the arm back and forth is a modified isometric-isotonic-type exercise. By working the biceps on the front of the arms against the triceps on the back of the arm, you increase its strength.

The strength and size of a muscle are directly related to putting a load on a muscle. Moving a muscle back and forth rapidly without putting a load on it will not increase its size. In the interest of maintaining muscle mass, a combination of isotonic-isometric exercise is useful. It's important not to overdo them. They can be done without overtensing of the muscle. Remember, they can make the muscle sore if you haven't done them in the past. Examples of these exercises are closing the hand, extending the fingers, tensing and relaxing the leg muscles, contracting and relaxing the abdominal muscles, and a large variety of other exercises. For a more detailed discussion of a variety of exercises that you could employ in such a system, see my earlier book, *Stay Youthful and Fit.*

Individuals who wish to prevent weight gain or eliminate excess fat deposits are advised to avoid the use of alcohol. Alcohol is a rich source of calories. Through its action on circulation, a process called "sludging," which involves the sticking together of the red blood cells, it can actually impair the delivery of oxygen to the cells. The addition of calories at the same time the available oxygen is diminished is a natural setup for stimulating the cell to use the fat-formation pathway. This may be one explanation why individuals who drink alcohol tend to develop excess fat deposits. Their alcohol will be stimulating fat synthesis as opposed to using the energy circle. Beyond these considerations, alcohol decreases will power, stimulates the appetite, and often results in overeating at a time when the body is least equipped and least likely to use these calories in any energy-expending activities.

Very often a successful weight-control program will be more successful if one employs the buddy system. That means finding one or more people who are interested in the same thing. Talk to to them about it and compare your success and your program. This is useful for both diet and exercise programs. A number of organizations where people get together and gain group support for weight-control programs have been successful. They encourage an individual to stay on the diet. The same is true for exercise efforts. Exercising with someone else helps make it more interesting and keeps you active on the day you might feel less motivated and less inclined to keep it up. Also helpful are regular and frequent checkups on the progress being made. Those individuals lucky enough to have an interested physician who will check their progress frequently will gain considerable additional benefit and motivation to continue the program.

Speaking of motivation, it is closely related to energy levels. The entire concept of metabolics is related to energy. If you have the proper nutritional dietary habits coupled with optimal living habits designed to maintain your bodily strength and vigor, your energy level will be high. Your energy will spill over into maintaining your motivation and make the whole system work better.

Metabolics is the concept that explains how your energy system works to support your basic life processes. Understand it and use it properly and you will have enough energy to make it unnecessary for you to indulge in the fads and gimmicks that victimize most overweight individuals. Beyond that, you will have the energy to make your life both longer and many times more enjoyable. It's more fun to have the energy to want to do things than it is to be tired and on a diet that robs you of your energy, decreases your inclination to engage in physical activity, decreases your ability to utilize energy, and sets up the vicious cycle of low energy and obesity. The scheme of nature allows the energies you get indirectly from the sun to be used to drive that wonderful machine, the human body. And, the methods for obtaining that energy and putting it all to use are based on the concepts of metabolics.

INDEX

(References to tables are printed in **boldface**)

acetate, active, 23–24, 128
  breakdown of pyruvic acid to, 43
acetic acid, 23, 89
acetoacetic acid, 59
acetone, formation of, 59
acetone breath, diabetic, 128
acidosis, 128
acid pepsin juice, hypoglycemia, 134
actin (protein), 26–27
Addison's disease, 120
adenine, 94
adenosine diphosphate (ADP), 21, 22,
  24, 27, 35, 40
  block diagram of, **22**
adenosine monophosphate (AMP), 21,
  22, 24
adenosine triphosphate (ATP), 21, 27,
  35, 39, 40, 42, 43, 44, 58, 59, 62,
  84, 88, 94
  block diagram of, 22
adrenal gland, diseases of, 137
adrenaline, 120–21
  blood glucose, low, 133
aerobic metabolism, 42
Aerospace Medical Center, 125
alanine, 68, 87–88, 91
  simple block diagram of, **69**
alcohol, 109
  assimilation of, 21–22, 98–99
  block diagram of, **97**
  blood glucose level, 101–2, 116–17
  calorie content of, 11, 97–98
  chemical composition, 55–56
  concentration in blood, **101**
  digestion of, 14
  and fatty liver, 111–12
  metabolism of, 99
  and weight control, 257
alcoholism, 98, 199
alcohol metabolism, flow diagram of,
  100
allopurinol (zyloprim), 95
alpha lipoprotein, 56
American Heart Association, 47
amino acids, 2, 67–68
  common pool of, 76, 87, 91, 104,
    107–8
  ketogenic nature of, 116
  manufacture of, 70–71
  metabolic function of, 27
  nonessential, **71**
  processing, flow diagram of, **90**
  and proteins, 11
  ten essential, **71**
amylose (ptyalin), 33, 34
anemia, 4–5

anxiety, 133
appetite-suppressing pills, 243
arginine, 71
ascorbic acid (vitamin C), 170–71
  block diagram of, **171**
  deficiency of, 171–72
  recommended daily allowance,
    172–73
  in some common foods, **175**
atherosclerosis, 10, 48, 56, 57, 66, 95
  and diabetes, 127, 129
Atkins, Dr., 212, 239, 240, 241

Banting, William, 238
Banting diet, 238
basal metabolism, 92–93
beans: in diet plan, 220–21
  protein in, **81**
beef: fat content, 50, 53–54
  protein source, **82**
beer, alcohol content, 98
Benedict, F. G., 230
beriberi, thiamine deficiency, 147
berries, protein in, 81
beta lipoproteins, 56
BHT (preservative), 12
bile, digestive function of, 15
bile salts, 66, 108
biotin, 168
  deficiency, 168–69
bladder, inflammation of, 126
blood: iron deficiency of, 200–201
  oxygenation of, 17–18
blood cells, white, formation of, 16
blood-fat level, in diabetes, 127
blood glucose, 33, 114–15
  levels of, 35, 40, 125
  production of, 44
blood glucose, hormones, balance
    illustration, **121**
blood glucose, low level, 5, 36, 117–18,
    120
  and carbohydrates, 9
  diet principles, 138
  production of, 135–36
  symptoms, 132–33
  see also hypoglycemia
blood hemoglobin test, for iron
    deficiency, 203
body heat, and proteins, 93
bone calcium, in fasting, 234 (see also
    calcium)
bone development, and vitamin D
    deficiency, 189
bone structure, 191–93

brain: alcohol, effect of, 100–101
    low-glucose level, effect of, 40
bread: diet plan, **221**
    protein content, 75
bread products, fat content, 53
breakfast, and reactive hypoglycemia,
    139
butter: calories in, 52
    fat content, 52

caffeine, 94
calcium, 191
    deficiency, 193
    flow chart, **192**
    in milk, 12
    in some common foods, **195**
    and vitamin D, 189, 193
calorie-restricted diets, blood glucose
    level, 125, 236
calories, 3, **247**
    and alcohol, 97–98
    as energy source, 20–21
    fat, stored as, 3–4
    men's daily usage, **248**
    requirements, average, 248–50
Calories Don't Count, 9, 171, 237, 238,
    242
carbohydrates:
    assimilation of, 21–22
    blood glucose level, 115
    daily need for, 32
    energy sources, 8–9
    defined, 28–29
    diabetic diet, 129
    packaging of, 33
    as protein-sparing energy source, 92
    restricted diet of, 8–9, 32, 40, 125
    source of, 69
carbon: elimination of, 24
    and fatty acids, 47
carbon dioxide, 18
    elimination of, 24
cells, body: active, 250
    alcohol, effect of, 102
    function of, 1–2
cellulose: chemical formation of, 31
    metabolic function, 8
cereal products, vitamin source, 77
cereals: diet plan, **221**
    fat content, 52
    protein in, **78**
cheese: fat content, 52
    protein in, **78**
chloride salts, 210
chlorophyll, 28
cholesterol, 55, 108
    and active acetate, 24
    content in some foods, **65**
    daily allowance of, 65
    egg yolks, content in, 70
    excess of, 110
    manufacture of, 64, 65
    processing of, 65–66

choline: amounts in food, **112**
    daily allowance, 112
    deficiency, 111–12
    defined, 111
chylomicron, 56
cirrhosis, of liver, 102, 111, 127
citric-acid cycle (Krebs cycle), 43
    block diagram of, **45**
cobalt, 204
coconut oil, fat content, 9–10, 52, 226
Coenzyme A (Co-A), 23, 24, 43, 44,
    59, 64, 107
cold cuts: fat content, 54
    protein source, 83
collagen, and ascorbic acid, 172
colon, function of, 18–19
copper, 204
corn, as starch, 31
corn oil, fat content, 52
cornstarch, 30–31
corn syrup, as single sugar, 32
corotene (provitamin), 176–77
cottage cheese, 139, 218
creatine phosphate (CP), 23, 24, 27
    block diagram of, **23**
cyanocobalamin (vitamin B₁₂), 163–64
    deficiency, 164–65
    recommended daily allowance, **165**
    in some common foods, **165**
cyanosis, in fad diets, 235–36
cystine, 80
cytochrome (protein), 26
cytochrome oxidase (enzyme), 26

Davis, Adelle, 29, 131, 144, 169, 178,
    197, 199
deamination, 87, 91
    block diagram of, **88**
desserts: baked, fat content, 54
    protein source, 83
dessert wine, alcoholic content, 98
dextrin, 21
dextrose (d-glucose), 29
diabetes, 5
    blood glucose level, 36, 124
    carbohydrates, 9
    coma, 59, 60
    defined, 123
    fat processing, 57
    fatty liver, 111
    lipotropic diet factor, 127
    mild, 124–25
    thirst, 126
    uncontrolled, glucose spill, 126
diabetic gangrene, 127
diarrhea, and double sugar intake, 38
diet, 3, 253–54
    for diabetic, 129–30
    vs. exercise, 251
    high fat, 239, 241
    protein content, adequate, 84
    protein deficiency, 5
    sodium loss, 211–12

diet (*cont'd*)
  vitamin fads, 143
diet, low-carbohydrate, 235, 237–42
  blood cholesterol level, 240–41
diet plan, 217–18, **218–19**
digestive problems, and protein intake, 85
disaccharide, 29
DNA (dioxiribonucleic acid), 95, 107
  and protein metabolism, 93–95
Dolomite tablets, 199
Dr. Atkins' Diet Revolution, 9, 171, 235, 237, 239, 242
Drinking Man's Diet, The, 242
dumping syndrome (low blood glucose), 136
duodenal ulcer, cause of, 13–14

eating habits, 253 (*see also* Diet)
eggs: diet plan, 221
  protein source, 78–79
  whites, protein source, 83
  yolk, fat and cholesterol content, 221
electrolytes, in diet, 11–12
energy: caloric source of, 20–21, 228–29
  hydrogen express mechanism, 26
  production of, 3, 20–23
  protein source of, 11
  use of, 26–27
energy levels: and active cells, 250–51
  and diet, 4–5
  and vitamins, 141
enzyme: defined, 23
  digestive function of, 15, 37
esophagus, 13
exercise, physical, 3, 250, 255–56
  and diabetes, 130
  fat processing, 63

fasting, and undernutrition, 230–31
fat (glycerol), 39
  and alcohol consumption, 102–3
  assimilation of, 21–22
  in blood vessels, 48
  caloric content, 47
  caloric source, 51
  in coconut oil, 10 (*see also* coconut oil)
  content in food, 9–10
  daily allowance, 54
  defined, 47–48
  diet intake, limitations, 226
  diet plan, 219
  energy source of, 59–61
  formation flow diagram, **62**
  glucose conversion, 233
  "hardened," 51
  in liver, diabetic, 127
  from mammal sources, 50
  monounsaturated, 9
  polyunsaturated, 9
  protein-sparing energy source, 92–93

saturated, 9, 49
  in stomach, role of, 55
  as triglyceride units, 58, 109
  unsaturated, 9
fat cells, defined, 56
fatigue: blood glucose, low-, 134–35
  diabetic symptom, 126–27
  measurement of, 142
  and oxygen supply, 5
fatty acids, 47, 48
  block diagram of, 48
  chemical composition of, 50
  as fat energy source, 58–59
  and glucose level, 116–17
  major, in human fat, **51**
  monounsaturated, 49
  and pituitary hormone, 120
  polyunsaturated, 49
  unsaturated, 49
feet, calcium needs, 194
fertility, and vitamin E, 182–83
fish: fat content, 53
  protein source, 81 (*see also* seafood)
  and shellfish, low-calorie, **252**
flavin, 25–26
folic acid, 166
  deficiency, 166–67
  recommended daily allowance, **167**
food, circulation of, 13
  flow diagram, **17**
Food and Drug Administration, The (FDA), 143, 167
  and vitamin E, 185
food intake, weight control, 251
fructose (mono-saccharide), 29
fruits: calories in, **252**
  diet plan, **225**
  fat content, 53
  metabolic processing of, 36
  protein in, 81

galactose (monosaccharide), 29
gelatin, as protein, 75, 83
glands, blood supply to, 16–18
glucagenic amino acids, **89**
glucogon, 121
gluconeogenesis, 116, 233
glucose (monosaccharide), 29
  in blood, 39 (*see also* blood glucose)
  as carbohydrate, 39, 105–6
  and diabetes, 123
  to glucose phosphate, block diagram of, **40**
  metabolism flow diagram for, **46**
  metabolism of, 89
  to phosphoglyceraldehyde, block diagram of, **41**
  sources of, 115
  tolerance test, 123
glucose phosphate, formation of, 39–40
gluten, low tolerance of, 227
gluten flour, protein source, 77, 80

glycerin, 41, 58
  defined, 47
  as glucose, 116
glycine, 68
  simple block diagram of, 69
glycogen (animal starch), 2, 31, 107,
    135–36
  formation of, 40
gout: causes: 94
  and diet, 95
  low-carbohydrate diet, 242
guanine, 94

Harvard Medical School, 240
Harvey, Dr. William, 238
heart attack, 66
  and diabetes, 127
heart disease, 47, 56–57, 95
  and carbohydrates, 9
  and fats, 221
  protein supplements, 85
heart muscle, alcoholic damage to, 102
hemoglobin, 26
hemorrhoids, 203
histidine, 71
honey: blood glucose level, 37
  as single sugar, 32
hormones: adrenal cortex, weight
    reduction, 120
  female, 63–64
  and muscle growth, 73
  as protein, 11
  sex, 108
hunger: blood glucose level, 254
  sensation of, 134
hydrogen: in kidneys, 26
  metabolic function of, 24–26
hydrogenation, partial, defined, 51
hydrogen express, 25, 42
  flow diagram of, 25
hypoglycemia: defined, 131–32
  functional, 136–37
  reactive, 136–37

inositol, 169
insulin, 86, 94
  blood glucose level, 118
  deficiency, 123
  defined, 67
  diabetic treatment, 128–29
  low level, 118–19
Inter-Society Commission on Heart
    Disease, 47, 65
intestine, small, function of, 14–15
intrinsic factor, iron needs, 201
iodine: deficiency, 207
  diet source, 206–7
  flow diagram, simple, 206
  thyroid function, 205–8
iron, 200–201
  deficiency, 200–201
  diet plan, 228
  in diet, 12

recommended daily allowance, **202**
  in some common foods, 203
isometric exercise, 256–57

*Journal of American Medical
    Association*, 132, 240

ketogenic amino acid, 89
ketone acetoacetic acid, 89
ketones, 59, 108, 239–40
  flow diagram, **61**
ketosis, 40
  in starvation, 234
Keys, Ancel, 235
kidneys: hemorrhage in, 112
  sodium processing, 211
Knisely, Melvin H., 102
Krook, Dr. Lennart, 194

lactose; in milk, 30
  intolerance of, 37
lamb: fat content, 50
  protein in, 83
laxatives, 243
lecithin, 112–13
  block diagram of, **113**
  defined, 111
Let's Eat Right to Keep Fit (Davis),
    29–30
leucine, 109
leukemia, 95
Levy, Magnus, 249
linoleic acid, 51
lipoprotein, and arterial fat deposits, 56
lipotropic deficiency, 112
lipotropic factor, 111
liquids, digestion of, 14
liver: cell damage from alcohol, 102
  diabetic damage, 127
  as fat processor, 56–57
  fatty, 111
  fatty acids, formation of, 65
  and glucose maintenance, 118
  iron source, 220
  and oxygenated blood flow, 18
  and vitamin A, 178–79
liver extract, and vitamin D, 189
liver glycogen, and blood glucose,
    115–16
lung disease, 4
Lutwak, Dr. Leo, 194
lymphatics, function of, 15–16

MacSiney, Terrance, 230
magnesium, 197
  deficiency, 197
  recommended daily allowance, **198**
  in some common foods, **198–99**
maltose (disaccharide), 29, 33–34,
    37–38
margarine, calories in, 7
mayonnaise, fat content, 53
meat: cholesterol content, 10

meat *(cont'd)*
 diet plan, 251–52
 protein source, 220
meat substitutes, diet plan, 220
megavitamin therapy, 143
melons, protein in, 81
metabolic map, **106**
metabolism: defined, 1
 simple flow diagram, **105**
milk, 34
 artificial, 79
 diet plan, 218
 protein in, 79–80
 purine free, 95
 skim, 12, 251
 whole, fat content, 53
milk substitutes, diet plan, 226–27
minerals, in diet, 11
minimum daily requirements (MDR),
 see under names of vitamins
mono-di-tri-glyceride, block diagram
 of, 49
monosaccharide (carbohydrate), 28–29
muscle building, 70
muscle maintenance, 246
mushrooms, protein in, 81
myoglobin, 201
myosin (protein), 26–27
 in animal muscle, 81

National Institutes of Health, 47
niacin: deficiency, 154
 recommended daily allowance, **155**
 in some common foods, **156–57**
 vitamin B-complex, 153–54
nicotinamide adeninedinucleotide
 (NAD), 25, 42, 58, 88, 141
nitrogen: in air, 69
 negative balance, 91
 in protein metabolism, 91–92
 in soil, 70
nuts, protein source, 83, **84**

obesity, 237
 blood glucose, low, 134
 causes of, 3
 diet, fat content, 51
 prevention of, 245–46, 251
 thyroid hormone, 208
oleic acid, 51
olive oil, fat content, 52
Olson, Dr. Robert, 183, 184
osteoporosis (porous bones), 194
oxaloacetic acid (OAA), 43, 44, 45,
 59, 61, 107
oxygen: fat processing, 63
 metabolic function of, 20
 purpose of, 13
oxygen level, alcohol effect on, 102

PABA, 167
pancreas, tumor of, 137
pancreatic juice, 34

pantothenic acid (vitamin B), 23,
 158–59
 deficiency, 159
Pauling, Linus, 173
pellagra, 153, 154
pentoses, in cell function, 31
pepsin, digestive function, 13–14
peptidases (enzymes), 86
peridontal disease, 194
Peter Bent Brigham hospital, 240
Peyronie's disease, 184–85
phosphate, 107
 as energy compounds, 21
phosphoglyceraldehyde (PGA), 41,
 58, 64, 107, 109
phosphorus, 196
 recommended daily allowance, 196
 and vitamin D, 189
pituitary gland: blood glucose level,
 high, 125
 blood glucose level, low, 137
pituitary hormone, blood glucose,
 119–21
pituitary tumor, hormone secreting, 125
polypeptide, 67
polysaccharide (poly sugar), 30
polyuria, 126
pork: fat content, 50, 54
 protein in, 83
 thiamine source, 220
potassium, 210
 in body, 12
 in diet, 215
potatoes, as starch, 31
poultry: diet plan, 220
 fat content, 53
 protein source, 82
protein, 2, 108
 assimilation of, 21–22
 from body secretions, 87
 coefficient of digestibility, 74
 daily adult requirements, 10
 diet plan, 219
 as energy supply, 68
 excess of, 73–74
 fat, conversion to, 73
 kinds of, 5–6
 muscle building, 72–73
 powders, 84
 processing of, 86–87
 quality of, 41–42
 recommended daily allowance, 72, 84
 supplements, 85, 113
 and undernutrition, 231–32
psychological behavior, and fad diets,
 236
purine, 94
pyridoxine (B₆), 161–62
 recommended daily allowance, **162**
pyrimidine bases, 95
pyruvic acid, 41
 to acetate, block diagram of, **44**
 to active acetate, 45

pyruvic acid (*cont'd*)
    block diagram of, **42**
    to oxaloacetic acid, block diagram
        of, **43**
    production of, 42–43

riboflavin (pigmented vitamin), 150–51
    deficiency, 150–51
    recommended daily allowance, **151**
    in some common foods, **151–52**
ribo-nucleic acid (RNA), 27, 107
    block diagram of, 96
    and protein metabolism, 93–95
ribosomes, 27
rickets, 189
Rickman, Dr. Frank, 240

safflower oil, fat content, 52
St. Louis School of Medicine, 183, 184
saliva, digestive function of, 13
salt: body needs for, 210–11
    diet plan, restricted, 85, 227
    and undernutrition, 232
saturated, unsaturated fats, block
        diagram, 50 (*see also* fat)
seafood, protein in, **81** (*see also* fish)
sex drive, and undernourishment, 235
sodium, 210–11
    diet, low-, 213
    foods high in, **214**
    foods moderately high in, **214**
    in meat, 213
    retention, 211
    in salt, 11–12
sodium chloride, sources, 213
sodium hydroxide, 212–13
soybeans, protein content, 80, 215
spirits, amount of yielding ½ ounce
        of alcohol, **98**
starch: block diagram of, **31**
    metabolism of, 31
    raw, digestion of, 34
starvation, 95
    blood glucose, low, 135
Stay Youthful and Fit (Lamb), 257
steroid hormones, 66
Stillman diet (water diet), 240
Stone, Irwin, 173
sucrose, 37–38

sugar: absorption by intestines, 35
    blood (*see* blood glucose)
    and protein, lack of, 77
    single, 35–36
sugar, double, 35
    block diagram of, **30**
    formation of, 30–31
sulfur, formation of, 23

thiamine, 145–46, 222–23
    recommended daily allowance, **147**
    in some common foods, **148–49**
thyroid: iodine intake, 205–8
    and obesity, 242–43
triglycerides, 48–50

urea, 18, 87, 89
    block diagram of, **88**
uric acid, 94–95

veal, protein source, 82
vegetables: caloric content, 53, **252**
    diet plan, **223–25**
    protein source, 75–76, 80
vitamin A, 176–77, 223
    deficiency, 177–79
    recommended daily allowance, **180**
vitamin B$_6$ (*see* pyridoxine)
vitamin B$_{12}$ (*see* cyanocobalamin)
vitamin C (*see* ascorbic acid)
vitamin D, 188–89, 193
    recommended daily allowance, 190
vitamin E, 182–83, 186, 221
    recommended daily allowance, **185**
vitamin K, 187

water, 7–8, 24, 210–12
weight, 73, 120, 128 (*see also* obesity)
    gaining, 4, 254–55
*What You Need to Know About Food
    and Cooking for Health*, 52
wheat, protein source, 77
wine, table, alcoholic content, 98
women, caloric usage, 247

xanthine, 94

yogurt, 219

76 77 10 9 8 7 6 5 4 3 2